Gastroenterology and Hepatology.
The next Millenium

John Libbey Eurotext
127, avenue de la République
92120 Montrouge
Tél. : 01 46 73 06 60

John Libbey and Company Ltd
13, Smiths Yard, Summerley Street
London SW18 4HR, England
Tel. : 1 947 27 77

John Libbey CIC
Via L. Spallanzani, 11
00161, Rome, Italie
Tel. : 06 862 289

© John Libbey Eurotext, 1998
ISBN : 2-7420-0232-4

Il est interdit de reproduire intégralement ou partiellement le présent ouvrage - loi du 11 mars 1957 - sans autorisation de l'éditeur.

Gastroenterology and Hepatology. The next Millenium

Edited by
G.N.J. Tytgat
G.J. Krejs

Postgraduate Course 1998
Vienna, September 5

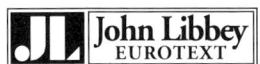

Contents

Presidential letter 1998
J.P. Galmiche IX

Oncology. Screening and surveillance

Molecular carcinogenesis in the gastrointestinal tract
Ph. Quirke 3

Molecular genetics in gastroenterology and hepatology. Where are we and where are we going?
P. Ferenci 5

Current, potential and future prospects for imaging modalities
R.J.H. Hammett, D.L. Carr-Locke 13

Pharmacology in hepatology and gastroenterology in the next Millenium

What is to be expected in acid related disorders: acid control and *Helicobacter pylori*
G. Sachs, J.M. Shin, M. Besançon, N. Lambrecht, D. Scott, D. Weeks, D. Melle, K. Melchers 25

Can cholesterol gallstones be prevented?
M.C. Carey 37

Drug therapy of Crohn's disease in the year 1998
C. van Montfrans, S.J.H. van Deventer 45

What should the clinician know about the cytochromes P450 system?
J.-P. Benhamou 59

The esophagogastric junction

What causes transient lower esophageal sphincter relaxations?
R.H. Holloway 67

The role of *Helicobacter pylori* in gastroesophageal reflux disease
P. Malfertheiner, C. Gerards 77

Inflammation and intestinal metaplasia of cardia and gastroesophageal junction
E. Solcia 89

Proton pump inhibitors or laparoscopic antireflux surgery?
L. Lundell 93

Progress in functional disorders

Functional disorders of the upper gastrointestinal tract. New concepts
R.H. Hunt, E.L. Fallen, M.V. Kamath, A.R.M. Upton, G. Tougas 105

Progress in functional disorders: functional lower intestinal disease
E.A. Mayer 111

List of contributors

Benhamou J.-P., Hôpital Beaujon, Clichy, France.

Besançon M., UCLA and Wadsworth VA Hospital, Los Angeles, CA USA.

Carey M.C., Brigham and Women's Hospital/Harvard Medical School, Boston, USA.

Carr-Locke D.L., Division of Gastroenterology, Brigham and Women's Hospital, Harvard Medical School, Boston, USA.

Fallen E.L., Division of Gastroenterology, Department of Medicine, McMaster University Medical Centre, Hamilton, Ontario L8N 3Z5, Canada.

Ferenci P., Department of Internal Medicine IV, Gastroenterology and Hepatology, University of Vienna, A 1090 Vienna, Austria.

Gerards C., Klinik für Gastroenterologie, Hepatologie und Infektiologie Otto von Guericke Universität, D-39120 Magdeburg, Germany.

Holloway R.H., Department of Gastrointestinal Medicine, Royal Adelaide Hospital, Adelaide, South Australia.

Hunt R.H., Division of Gastroenterology, Department of Medicine, McMaster University Medical Centre, Hamilton, Ontario L8N 3Z5, Canada.

Kamath M.V., Division of Gastroenterology, Department of Medicine, McMaster University Medical Centre, Hamilton, Ontario L8N 3Z5, Canada.

Lambrecht N., UCLA and Wadsworth VA Hospital, Los Angeles, CA USA.

Lundell L., Department of Surgery, Sahlgrenska University Hospital, S-413 45 Göteborg, Sweden.

Malfertheiner P., Klinik für Gastroenterologie, Hepatologie und Infektiologie Otto von Guericke Universität, D-39120 Magdeburg, Germany.

Mayer E.A., UCLA School of Medicine, Los Angeles, CA 90024 USA.

Melchers K., Byk Gulden, Konstanz, Germany.

Melle D., UCLA and Wadsworth VA Hospital, Los Angeles, CA USA.

Quirke Ph., Leeds University, Leeds LS 2 9JT, UK.

Sachs G., UCLA and Wadsworth VA Hospital, Los Angeles, CA USA.

Scott D., UCLA and Wadsworth VA Hospital, Los Angeles, CA USA.

Shin J.M., UCLA and Wadsworth VA Hospital, Los Angeles, CA USA.

Solcia E., Department of Pathology, University of Pavia and IRCCS Policlinico San Matteo, Pavia, Italy.

Tougas G., Division of Gastroenterology, Department of Medicine, McMaster University Medical Centre, Hamilton, Ontario L8N 3Z5, Canada.

Upton R.M., Division of Gastroenterology, Department of Medicine, McMaster University Medical Centre, Hamilton, Ontario L8N 3Z5, Canada.

van Deventer J.H., Laboratory of Experimental Internal Medicine, Academic Medical Center, Amsterdam, the Netherlands.

van Montfrans C., Laboratory of Experimental Internal Medicine, Academic Medical Center, Amsterdam, the Netherlands.

Weeks D., UCLA and Wadsworth VA Hospital, Los Angeles, CA USA.

Presidential letter 1998

On behalf of the Governing Board of our Society, I am especially happy and honoured to welcome you to this Post-Graduate Course organised by our Society on the occasion of the World Congress of Gastroenterology (Vienna, September 5, 1998). This year our Post-Graduate Course has been prepared by Prof. G.J. Krejs, the President of the World Congress, and Prof. G.N.J. Tytgat.

The programme is of outstanding interest and involves an impressive International Faculty. According to a now well-established practice, this Course is accompanied by the publication of this monograph including the full papers corresponding to the different topics discussed. This monograph is the 5th of a series, which is now an important part of our educational programme.

This occasion also gives me the opportunity to announce two other important Courses to be held during the coming year. The first will be organised by Prof. Malfertheiner and Prof. Butruk in Magdeburg (November 13-14) and is aimed at bridging Gastroenterology between the East and the West of Europe. Finally, another important Course will take place in Paris on July 1999, devoted to "Inflammatory Bowel Disease" (Dir: Prof. J.F. Colombel) and "Neuro-endocrine tumors of the gut" (Dir: Prof. M. Mignon in conjunction with the ENET group).

We are confident that such continuous efforts will be increasingly attractive to gastroenterologists, surgeons and scientists working in the field of Gastroenterology and Endoscopy in Europe. Because we need your support to achieve all these goals, I strongly invite you to join the Society and enjoy all the advantages and privileges of membership.

Finally, I would like to invite you to the General Assembly that will be held during this Course since important decisions will be taken, especially the election of the next President.

J.P. Galmiche
President of EAGE

Oncology.
Screening and surveillance

Molecular carcinogenesis in the gastrointestinal tract

Ph. Quirke

Leeds University, Leeds LS 2 9JT, UK

The gastrointestinal tract is the most frequent site for tumour formation and cancer death in Europe. Due to the case of access to the frequently affected sites and the work of gastrointestinal pathologists and their clinical colleagues much is known about the pathways that lead to their formation. The molecular basis of these lesions are the best understood of all the human cancers especially in the colorectum. Many of the tumours share the most important lesions in tumour suppressor genes and oncogenes with frequent involvement of p53 and Ki-ras and less frequent involvement of DNA repair genes. To date colorectal cancer has benifited most from such knowledge and owing to limited time will be used as an example of what is likely to happen in the other tumours.

The development of colorectal cancer can occur by at least 7 pathways. The molecular basis of FAP, HNPCC, Peutz-Jeghers and Juvenile polyposis have now been elucidated. The other pathways of the sporadic polypoid adenoma-carcinoma sequence, the flat adenoma-carcinoma sequence and the ulcerative colitis-carcinoma sequence are also partially understood.

The apc tumour suppressor gene on 5q.21 encodes a 15 exon gene. apc interacts with the Wnt/wingless signalling system, the E-cadherin pathway and the cytoskeleton. Wild type apc binds to beta-catenin targeting it for destruction. Mutations of apc leads to an accumulation of beta catenin, its transfert to the nucleus and gene activation when the beta-catenin-hTcf-4 complex binds to DNA. Mutations of apc also lead to disorganisation of the microtubular system. apc lesions cause abnormal proliferation, migration and cell death leading to adenoma formation. FAP can be diagnosed by mutation detection usually in the mutation cluster region or the protein truncation test.

HNPCC is caused defects in h-MSH-2, h-MLH-1, h-PMS-1, h-PMS-2 or GTBP. The proteins produced by these genes recognize damage to DNA caused by DNA slippage. h-MSH-2 identifies the damage initiating the formation of the complex with the other DNA repair genes. h-MSH-2 lesions are most frequent followed by h-MLH-1. Not all cases link to the known DNA repair genes. Defects of DNA repair leads to microsatellite instability (MI). The presence of MI in adenomas appears to be the most sensitive indicator of HNPCC in the absence of sequencing the genes. Mutations are spread throughout the genes making molecular diagnosis difficult. Immunocytochemistry for loss of the same gene product in cancers in different members of the family may yield a new rapid method of identifying h-MSH-2 or h-MLH-1 HNPCC families.

In sporadic carcinoma there are usually more than 5 lesions. The earliest lesion is inactivation of apc, hypomethylation of genes followed by bcl-2 overexpression. Ki-ras mutations develop in up to 40% of adenomas, accompanied by abnormalities of telomerase, and loss of 18q in the area of DCC. At the adenoma-carcinoma interface abnormalities of p53 arise leading to failure to recognise DNA damage, cell cycle arrest/repair or apotosis and abnormal centrosome function. This leads to a rapid propagation of DNA damage and the development of chromosomal aneuploidy. In 15% of sporadic carcinomas MI can be found suggesting defects in DNA repair pathways occur. This is usually seen in right sided diploid cancers. Patients with multiple cancers have a higher frequency of MI and these individuals have a 5 fold excess risk of developing a metachronous cancer and have a better prognosis. They are usually due to inactivation of h-MLH-1 gene rather than h-MSH-2 (ratio of cases 14:1) possibly by methylation of the h-MLH-1 promoter. It is now possible to identify such lesions by immunocytochemistry with a 95-100% accuracy. A large number of other lesions occur after invasion affecting invasion and metastasis but these are not as well characterised.

In the flat-adenoma-carcinoma pathway there are changes in the expression of p53 when compared to polypoid adenomas but to date no other differences have been reported.

In ulcerative colitis there is earlier overexpression of p53 and there may be a reduction in Ki-ras mutation but other tumour suppressor genes appear to show similar abnormalities to sporadic carcinoma.

Molecular genetics in gastroenterology and hepatology. Where are we and where are we going?

P. Ferenci

Department of Internal Medicine IV, University of Vienna, 1090 Vienna, Austria

Modern techniques of molecular biology unraveled the genetic background of many diseases. Three new diseases causing mutations of previously unknown genes are reported weekly. It has been estimated that the full human genome will be decoded within the next few years. These discoveries help us to understand disease mechanisms, to design new treatments and to diagnose diseases at an early stage. The application of molecular genetics in clinical medicine is just emerging.

Tools of molecular genetic analysis

DNA-polymorphisms

One of the most important tools of molecular genetics is the ability to visualize sequence differences directly in DNA. When studied in the context of a population, these differences in DNA sequences are called polymorphisms; they may occur in coding regions (exons) or noncoding regions of genes (for review: [1]). Such DNA-polymorphisms are inherited according to the Mendelian rules. If a DNA-polymorphisms has no effect on gene function, the resulting variations in physico-chemical properties of genomic DNA or of the gene product are designated alleles (*i.e.* blood groups). Changes in the nucleotide sequence which are associated with differences (loss or gain) in function are mutations.

The value of highly variable DNA sequences as genetic markers rests on straightforward principles. Every person carries two copies of each chromosome except the sex chromosomes. If a DNA polymorphism is to be useful in analyzing the transmission of the two chromosomes in a family, then the DNA copies at the polymorphic site of the person under study must be different in the two chromosomes. The likelihood that a given person will have different DNA sequences at the polymorphic site directly determines the usefulness of that site in genetic studies.

Chromosomal sites at which the DNA sequences can have many alternative forms are thus ideal sites for genetic markers. At these sites, a person is most likely to carry two alternative DNA sequences, accurately marking the two alternative chromosomes. In the human genome, the sites that have the properties most favorable to such extensive variation include a repetition of the same short DNA sequence a variable number of times. Such sequences are called tandem-repeat sequences (microsatellites). A DNA sequence with such variation may be as short as two base pairs or as long as several hundred base pairs. Highly variable sequences of this type are well distributed throughout the length of every human chromosome. When tandemly repeated sequences are replicated during cell division, the number of repeats can change.

Methods to detect DNA-polymorphisms

Restriction fragment length polymorphism (RFLP) analysis

DNA-polymorphisms can be detected by variations in the size of DNA fragments obtained after digestion with restriction enzymes (for review: [2, 3]). Restriction enzymes cut DNA-strands at highly specific sites (restriction site). A variation in the nucleotide sequence may result in the loss or the creation of a new restriction site or in the length of the DNA-fragment between existing restriction sites. Thus, the length (and eventually also the number) of the restriction fragment(s) will be different. DNA fragments separated by PAGE can be detected by DNA probes specific for the gene. If the gene is unknown, polymorphic markers flanking the unknown gene can be used. The RFLP pattern is specific for every individual tested. By employing various restriction enzymes and DNA-probes, multiple RFLP's for a given gene can be obtained. By this approach, both the paternal and the maternal gene can be "reconstructed". If both genes (haplotypes) have different allele patterns which are also different within members of the family, the pattern of its inheritance can be traced.

By DNA linkage analysis inheritance of a disease can be studied even if the gene/and or the mutation are unknown. Precondition for DNA-linkage analysis is the availability of an index patient (in whom the disease was diagnosed by standard phenotypic criteria) and both of his/her parents for testing. Limitations of DNA linkage analysis are the lack of informative allelic markers within the family and the presence of cross-overs within the region of interest. DNA-linkage analysis is time consuming and can only be applied in selected families. The importance of RFLP analysis is the localization of an unknown gene to a distinct part of a chromosome. This information is needed for the identification of a disease gene by a variety of methods.

Direct mutation analysis

Direct sequencing

New technologies allow automated DNA-sequence analysis of large portions of a gene. Thereby points mutations, deletions, inversions and other changes in the nucleotide sequence can be visualized. However, direct sequencing of the whole gene plays yet no role in clinical medicine. A more practical approach is first to screen the gene of interest for possible mutation by haplotype analysis or by single-strand conformation polymorphism analysis. Those samples showing a shift of one or both bands or unusual haplotypes can then be sequenced to identify the exact mutation. This approach is quite useful as research tool, but impractical for clinical diagnosis.

PCR-based detection of known mutations

A variety of approaches are commonly used to detect mutations. One of the simplest takes advantage of the base-sequence specificity of restriction endonucleases. These enzymes recognize precise sequences of four to eight bases and cut double-stranded DNA only at these sites. A mutation at such a site will prevent the enzyme from cutting there; conversely, a mutation may result in the creation of a new enzyme-recognition site and lead to cutting where it normally should not occur. To detect the mutation, DNA surrounding the site of potential mutation is amplified by the polymerase chain reaction (PCR), the product is incubated with the restriction enzyme, and then the DNA is analyzed by electrophoresis. If the enzyme cuts, two fragments will result; otherwise there will be a single fragment. The presence or absence of the mutation can be inferred, depending on whether the mutation creates or destroys an enzyme-recognition site.

The other scheme for detecting mutations, is based on the specificity of the PCR reaction itself. A PCR primer is designed that ends right at the site of a potential mutation. If the primer is homologous to the wild-type sequence, it will amplify only the wild-type sequence in conjunction with another primer some distance away in the gene. The wild-type primer will not amplify mutant DNA, however. Conversely, a primer that is homologous to the mutant sequence will amplify only mutant DNA. If the PCR is carried out with both sets of primers in separate reactions, the presence or absence of mutant and wild-type sequences can easily be determined. Here multiple sequences can be assayed simultaneously in a single sample, as long as the sizes of the PCR products from each segment differ.

The direct determination of mutations is independent of family analysis. There is no need to test an index patients with the disease. PCR-based mutation assays can be automated and thus allow mass screening. Several mutation assays are commercially available now (see *table I*).

Table I. Most common hereditary diseases in digestive disease with identified mutations

	Disease	Gene	Chromosome	Commercial test
Colon cancer	FAP	APC	5	Protein assay
	NHPCC	MLH1	3	In preparation
		MSH2	2	
		Others		
	Other polyposis syndromes	Multiple		
Liver disease	Hereditary hemochromatosis	HFE	6	Cys282Tyr PCR-test
	Wilson disease	ATP 7B	13	
	α1-antitrypsin deficiency	α1-antitrypsin	14	Electrophoresis, Isoelectric focuing
	Disorders of bilirubin metabolism	Multiple		
	Disorders of organic anion transporters	Multiple	5	
Pancreatic disease	Cystic fibrosis	CFTR	7	DeltaAF508 mutant protein

Target populations for molecular genetic testing

Subjects with symptomatic phenotypic disease

In a patient with a hereditary disease (diagnosed by phenotypic criteria; *i.e.* polyposis coli), molecular genetic analysis strengthens the final diagnosis in the absence of other affected family members. Precise identification of the mutation is extremely helpful in screening the family of the index patient.

Family screening

Mutation analysis can replace other diagnostic tests to identify subjects at risk to develop the disease [4]. A negative test result in someone from a family in which affected relatives are known to have a disease-related mutation indicates a low risk of the disease. This can decrease anxiety and, for some diseases, reduce the frequency of periodic monitoring for early signs of the disease. The applicability and cost effectiveness of mutation analysis depends specific characteristics of the disease. For example, in FAP testing for APC mutations is superior to endoscopy in children and young adults, whereas endoscopy is more appropriate in older family members [5].

Patients with symptoms or diseases with a potential genetic background (*i.e.* patients with colon cancer at young age)

In general, definition of a diseases is based on typical symptoms. The presence of all symptoms is usually required for diagnosis. For example, diagnosis of hereditary hemochromatosis requires at least two affected family members. If a patient has no siblings, the diagnosis of hereditary hemochromatosis cannot be made. For other disease there are international diagnostic criteria (*i.e.* for HNPCC). In oligosymptomatic patients (who do not meet the diagnostic criteria) genetic tests may be useful to make the diagnosis [6].

Population screening

Mutation analysis to detect presymptomatic disease in the general population has not been tested so far. There are several conditions which limit the use of such tests for screening, the most important ones are the difficulties of interpretation of test results [7].

Interpretation of test results

Direct mutation analysis can yield three possible findings: the tested subject is either a homozygous or a heterozygous carrier of the mutation, or does not carry the mutation at all. The interpretation of each of these results has limitations.

Homozygous mutation carrier

In contrast to the phenotypic diagnosis of a disease, genotypic diagnosis in a healthy subject raises the question, whether tested subject will ever develop the disease. In most hereditary diseases there is no complete penetrance of the disease. In genetic hemochromatosis for example, 17% of Cys282Tyr (the typical mutation) homozygotes have no evidence of iron overload [8]. The same applies also for carriers of the breast cancer gene Brac 1 [9]. The fundamental difference is what recommendations are given. In a subject homozygous for genetic hemochromatosis life long voluntary blood donations may prevent development of cirrhosis. Thus counseling is quite simple. In subjects at risk to develop a life threatening cancer, however, there are no clear guidelines for prevention strategies. A young subject carrying mutations of the APC-gene but no colonic adenomas may undergo prophylactic colectomy, participate in a close endoscopic surveillance program or may receive chemoprevention with NSAID's. Thus, before a gene test is introduced to clinical medicine, such guidelines have to be formulated and validated by prospective trials. Before such guidelines are adopted, only first degree relatives of index cases should be tested. In other subjects, the limitations of mutation tests should be explained prior testing and an informed consent should be obtained.

Heterozygous mutation carrier

In this setting the most important question is, whether the tested subject is (and will remain) free of a disease or not. According Mendelian rules, subjects carrying a healthy (wild type) and a disease gene with autosomal recessive inheritance are healthy. This statement depends on the definition of a "normal" gene. The absence of a detectable mutation is not sufficient that the gene product of such a gene in functionally intact.

Compound heterozygotes

The gene not having the mutation may have a different (disease causing) one, which is simply not detected by the assay. Such compound heterozygotes may suffer from the disease (diagnosed by phenotypic criteria). Unfortunately this is not an exception but a general rule. In most inherited disease multiple different mutations of the affected gene are present (more than 450 in cystic fibrosis, more than 100 in Wilson disease [10]). Mutations may reflect a common ancestor and are enriched in certain populations but may be absent in others [11]. Thus, a test useful in Northern Europe may be quite useless in Southern Europe.

Loss of heterozygosity

Subjects with a normal and an abnormal gene without any apparent disease may undergo somatic mutations of the normal gene later in life. Such event may result in overt dysfunction of the gene product in the affected cells. This loss of heterozygosity is assumed to be one important event in cancerogenesis [12].

Subjects not carrying the mutation

As discussed before, a negative finding does not exclude disease, since other mutations of the gene may be present. Furthermore, gene defects may be due to mutation of other genes (*i.e.* mutation of promoters of mismatch repair genes results in hypermethylation of their genes products with impaired functional capacity).

Current recommendations for molecular genetic testing

– Formulation of an acceptable procedure for counseling subjects with a positive test before adopting a mutation test for clinical use.

– Identification of the population to be tested (1st degree relatives with the disease, subjects with phenotypic signs of the disease or general population).

– Prospective studies to compare sensitivity, specificity and cost effectiveness of genetic testing *versus* phenotypic screening.

– Informed consent prior testing.

References

1. Housman D. Human DNA-polymorhism. *N Engl J Med* 1995; 332: 318-9.
2. Korf B. Molecular Diagnosis (First of Two Parts). *N Engl J Med* 1995; 332: 1218-21.
3. Korf B. Molecular Diagnosis (Second of Two Parts). *N Engl J Med* 1995; 332: 1499-502.
4. Maier-Dobersberger Th, Rack S, Granditsch G, Korninger L, Steindl P, Mannhalter Ch, Ferenci P. Diagnosis of Wilson's disease in an asymptomatic sibling by DNA linkage analysis. *Gastroenterology* 1995; 109: 2015-8.
5. Cromwell DM, Moore RD, Brensinger JD, Petersen G, Bass E, Gardiella FM. Cost analysis of alternative approaches to colorectal screening in familial adenomatous polyposs. *Gastroenterology* 1998; 114: 893-901.
6. Lynch HT, Smyrk TC. Identifying hereditary colorectal cancer. *N Engl J Med* 1998; 338: 1537-8.
7. Giardiello FM, Brensinger JD, Petersen GM, *et al.* The use and interpretation of commercial APC gene testing for familial adenomatous polyposis. *N Engl J Med* 1997; 336: 823-7.
8. Crawford DHG, Jazwinska EC, Cullen LM, Powell L. Expression of HLA-linked hemochromatosis in subjects homozygous or heterozygous for the C282Y mutation. *Gastroenterology* 1998; 114: 1003-8.
9. Struewing JP, Hartge P, Wacholder S, *et al.* The risk of cancer associated with specific mutations of BRCA1 and BRCA2 among Askhenazi Jews. *N Engl J Med* 1997; 336: 1401-8.
10. Maier-Dobersberger Th, Ferenci P, Polli C, Balac P, Dienes HP, Kaserer K, Datz C, Vogel W, Gangl A. Detection of the His1069Gln mutation in Wilson disease by a rapid polymerase chain reaction. *Ann Intern Med* 1997; 127: 21-6.
11. Piperno A, Sampietro M, Pietrangelo A, *et al.* Heterogeneity of hemochromatosis in Italy. *Gastroenterology* 1998; 114: 996-1002.
12. Jen J, Kim H, Piantadosi S, *et al.* Allelic loss of chromosome 18q and prognosis in colorectal cancer. *N Engl J Med* 1994; 331: 213-21.

Current, potential and future prospects for imaging modalities

R.J.H. Hammett, D.L. Carr-Locke

Division of Gastroenterology, Brigham and Women's Hospital, Harvard Medical School, Boston, USA

This paper will deal mainly with the current and potential uses of new modalities such as virtual colonoscopy in screening for colorectal cancer. However, it is important to make note of advances in other imaging techniques that will play a role in screening and surveillance of malignancies elsewhere in the gastrointestinal tract. In particular, a number of techniques that have been available for some time are finding new applications in the surveillance of high risk patients in conditions such as Barrett's esophagus, gastric carcinoma and rectal carcinoma, and these will be discussed briefly.

Current screening practices

Esophageal carcinoma

Current recommendations regarding surveillance of Barrett's esophagus (four quadrant biopsies at 1 cm intervals) are not easily followed in daily clinical practice, and controversy continues regarding the management of high grade dysplasia in this setting. Screening and surveillance for esophageal cancer is at present dependent on endoscopic techniques, but, as discussed below, these techniques are being refined to improve sensitivity.

Gastric carcinoma

Endoscopic imaging is the mainstay of screening programs in areas with high rates of gastric cancer. The effectiveness of chromoendoscopy, ultra-high magnification endoscopy and virtual endoscopy in detection of early gastric lesions is currently being evaluated. Although advances in imaging technology are rapid, it is likely that for the foreseeable future endoscopy will continue to form the basis for screening programs in countries such as Japan where gastric cancer is common.

Pancreatic carcinoma

Patients at higher risk of developing malignancy, such as those with chronic pancreatitis and familial cancer syndromes, are most likely to benefit from screening programs for pancreatic cancer. Advances in EUS, CT and MRCP all offer hope for effective evaluation of pancreatic pathology, although at this stage data are not available on the effects of such imaging on morbidity and mortality.

Hepatocellular carcinoma

The high incidence of hepatocellular carcinoma in parts of the world where hepatitis B is endemic has necessitated development of screening programs involving regular ultrasound and measurement of α feto-protein in at risk populations. The benefits of such screening have not been shown to be cost-effective in parts of the world in which hepatitis B is not endemic, but these strategies are commonly utilized in clinical practice.

Biliary carcinoma

Parts of South America, the Indian subcontinent and South-East Asia have a higher incidence of carcinoma of the biliary tree than that seen in Europe and the United States. Numerous serum markers have been studied in these groups to attempt to identify a suitable screening tools, with little success thus far. Advances in imaging technology (MRCP, virtual endoscopy) in Europe and the United States have improved visualization of anatomical defects in the biliary tree, but are unlikely to be suitable tools for screening programs in other parts of the world. Suitable molecular and biochemical markers are more likely to offer realistic screening and surveillance methods in these areas.

Colorectal carcinoma

In the United States, implementation of screening recommendations has often been hampered by financial considerations concerning reimbursement by third party payers until this year when medicare and other insurers approved coverage for screening. Worldwide, availability of endoscopists and equipment has been more important.

Colorectal cancer is the second leading cause of cancer death in the United States, accounting for 55,000 deaths in 1997. The lifetime risk for development of CRC in an average risk individual has been estimated to be approximately 6%.

Despite the fact that 30% of all colonic malignancies occur proximal to the splenic flexure, flexible sigmoidoscopy rather than colonoscopy is the most common form of colonic imaging in average risk patients. Current screening programs using fecal occult blood and flexible sigmoidoscopy will miss a proportion of patients with proximal lesions. As it is expected that 25% of adults will have colonic polyps at age 50, and given that there is a well-documented adenoma-carcinoma sequence in the colon, it is likely that the number of patients with potentially malignant colonic lesions is not insignificant. Thus, in the United States, there is currently a need for cheap and reliable alternatives to current screening modalities, or legislative changes that will enable more widespread use of techniques capable of imaging the entire colon.

Current recommendations for screening for colorectal cancer in the United States are summarized in *table I* and *II*. The guidelines do not apply to individuals with a first degree relative aged less than 60 with CRC, nor to Familial Polyposis or Hereditary Non-Polyposis Coli Carcinoma patients, in whom colonoscopy is indicated at regular intervals.

The role of barium enema in screening for CRC is not well established despite its inclusion in these guidelines. Indeed, as shown in the National Polyp Study [1], the sensitivity fo double-contrast barium enema for detecting large polyps is only 50%. It is estimated that the cost of screening for CRC using current guidelines is approximately $20,000 per year of life saved.

Table I. 1997 Guidelines for colorectal cancer screening in average-risk persons (age > 50 years)

Agency for health care policy and research
- Annual fecal occult blood test.
- Flexible sigmoidoscopy every 5 years.
- Combination of above.
- Double contrast barium enema every 5-10 years.
- Colonoscopy every 10 years.

American Cancer Society

- Annual fecal occult blood test plus flexible sigmoidoscopy every 5 years.
- Double contrast barium enema every 5-10 years.
- Colonoscopy every 10 years.

Patients and physicians choose one of the options.
The options are not equal with regard to efficacy, cost or risk.
The advantage of multiple options is to provide increased choice to patients, physicians and payers.

Table II. High-risk screening for colorectal cancer

- Family history of colorectal cancer or adenoma in first degree relative diagnosed at age < 60 years or two first degree relatives with either cancer or adenomas: colonoscopy every 3-5 years; beginning at age 40, or 10 years younger than the youngest affected relative, whichever is first.
- Women with breast cancer; same screening as average risk women.

Potential practice with current modalities

Chromoendoscopy

The use of dyes and stains to enhance endoscopic imaging is not a new technique and has been used for some time in parts of the world where upper GI malignancies are common. Recognition of the increased incidence of adenocarcinoma of the esophagus in the last twenty years has focused attention on methods of detecting early carcinoma in the esophagus in Europe and the United States. Adenocarcinoma has risen from 0.8-3.7% of esophageal cancers in series between 1926-1996, to 54%-68% in series between 1978-1992. The reasons underlying the changing incidence of this histological subtype of esophageal cancer remain unclear.

Lugol's iodine utilizes the reduced glycogen content of glandular and carcinomatous epithelia to distinguish potentially malignant tissue from squamous epithelium in the esophagus. Toluidine Blue stains nuclei and may preferentially identify malignant and inflammatory tissue as a result of a greater nuclear cytoplasmic ratio.

Use of both of these agents may facilitate the diagnosis of early esophageal carcinoma [2, 3] and improve preoperative assessment of extent of disease [2, 4].

Both agents have improved the identification of early stage occult cancer in screening programs for high risk patients [3, 5], but yield false positive staining due to acute and chronic inflammation [6] and are insensitive for dysplasia [6].

Methylene blue has been used alone, or in combination with Congo Red to identify intestinal metaplasia and minute synchronous gastric cancer [7]. The reported sensitivity of methylene blue alone in intestinal metaplasia is 80-98% and its specificity is 89-99%.

Other dyes have been used in the stomach and colon and their properties and uses are listed in *table III*.

Chromoendoscopy is a safe, cheap and well tolerated method of increasing the yield of screening for upper GI malignancy in high-risk individuals, and is rightly gaining more widespread acceptance.

Endoscopic ultrasound

Endorectal ultrasound has been shown to be superior to CT scan for local staging of rectal cancer and may be of use in surveillance of patients with rectal cancer as there is a high rate of local recurrence in these patients than in patients with colorectal cancer. The number of patients that would benefit from this surveillance remains to be determined, as does the cost effectiveness of EUS in this setting.

Table III. Commonly described stains and inks for endoscopic application

Stain	Mechanism of staining	Described uses
Lugol's iodine	Stains glycogen in non-keratinized squamous epithelia to brown	Esophageal squamous cell carcinoma Peptic esophagitis Barrett's esophagus
Methylene blue	Stains physiologically absorptive tissues blue	Intestinal metaplasia of stomach Gastric cancer Gastric metaplasia of duodenum
Toluidine blue	Stains the nuclei of malignant cells blue	Squamous cell carcinoma of esophagus and oropharynx
Congo red	pH indicator which turns from red to dark blue-black in the presence of acid at pH < 3.0	Map acid secretion of gastric mucosa in stomach and in ectopic locations Gastric cancer screen with methylene blue
Phenol red	pH indicator which turns from yellow to red during alkalinization from pH 6.8-8.4	Identification and mapping of urease production by *H. pylori* when administered with a urea solution
Indigo carmine	Non-absorbed stain highlights mucosal irregularities with blue contrast	Identification of inconspicuous mucosal lesions including polyps and dysplasia of the esophagus or colon
India ink	Submucosal injection to permanently label a location of the gut for future identification of the serosal or luminal aspect	Labeling locations of malignant polyps and other lesions or therapies for subsequent surveillance, intraoperative identification, or study of natural history
Indocyanine green	Parenteral dye used for cardiac and hepatic function studies Described as potentially benign tattooing agent	As for India ink

Magnetic resonance cholangiopancreatography

Since its inception MRCP has offered the promise of non-invasive diagnosis of biliary and pancreatic malignancy. At present there is conflicting data regarding its ability to distinguish between chronic inflammatory conditions such as chronic pancreatitis and sclerosing cholangitis and the malignancies that complicate such conditions. In cases where ERCP is not technically possible, MRCP offers non-invasive imaging with similar sensitivity to ERCP that can allow decisions regarding further treatment to be made with adequate information [10]. It is likely that MRCP will gain wider use in parts of the world in which it is available in providing screening and surveillance of patients at high risk of pancreatic or biliary malignancy.

Future techniques of screening of GI malignancies

New screening tools must be accurate, reliable, reproducible and cost-effective. They must also result in directly measurable benefits to patients in terms of morbidity and mortality, and ideally also provide improvements over current techniques in terms of patient tolerance and compliance. Data from well-designed controlled trials should be obtained prior to implementation of any screening strategy involving the technological advances described below.

Virtual endoscopy

The terms "virtual endoscopy" and "CT colography" refer to the technique whereby a computer dataset obtained when a patient undergoes a spiral CT is manipulated by computer software to enable presentation of graphic images similar to the view presented by direct endoscopy.

This technique has been used in both the upper and lower gastrointestinal tract, but appears to be more useful in detection of colonic pathology than in esophageal or gastric lesions.

Virtual colonoscopy was first shown to be a feasible means of detecting colonic lesions by Vining *et al.* [11]. It involves cleansing of the bowel with a standard bowel preparation regimen, insufflation of air or carbon dioxide into the colon using a standard enema tube, administration of intravenous glucagon, and acquisition of data by a helical CT using a 30-60 second single breath hold technique.

The captured data are stored in the form of a volume of information that must then be analyzed by a radiologist in such a way as to obtain sufficiently detailed views of the colon. The time required to produce a virtual reality rendering of the colonic lumen is a reflection of the size of the dataset specified by the radiologist, as is the degree of accuracy of the technique.

At present there are a number of problems with this procedure. The patient must undergo a bowel cleansing regimen similar to conventional colonoscopy, and insufficient cleansing of the bowel makes analysis of the resultant images difficult due to the higher false positive and false negative rate. Flat lesions are not well seen and potentially serious sessile lesions may well be missed using currently available technology. In addition, analysis of the dataset produced by the spiral CT is a time consuming procedure for the radiologist involved and is open to observer error. Data presented at DDW in 1997 and 1998 showed that the ability of virtual colonoscopy to detect colonic polyps is a reflection of polyp size, and that smaller polyps (< 1 cm) may well be missed by this technique.

The primary perceived benefits of virtual colonoscopy are 1) that it will be better tolerated by patients and 2) that it will have lower complication rates than conventional colonoscopy. At present data are unavailable to support these assumptions, and the fact that patients may need to undergo a second bowel cleansing regimen and a colonoscopy if polyps are seen on virtual colonoscopy, may well affect patient acceptance of the procedure.

Nevertheless, taking into consideration the problems mentioned above, virtual colonoscopy is an exciting prospect. The rapid advances in computer software and hardware that are continually occurring are likely to reduce data analysis times to levels where it will soon become feasible for virtual colonoscopy to be performed outside research settings. Indeed, automated analysis software has already been reported [12] and may eliminate the time consuming involvement of radiologists in the procedure. In addition, improvement in spiral CT scanner technology itself has resulted in the development of multi-detector scanners which will increase data acquisition speeds four-to six-fold. This will enable higher spatial resolution and hopefully better sensitivity and specificity.

At present the patient is only required in the radiology department for 15 minutes, and receives a radiation dose equivalent to two plain abdominal X-rays. This radiation exposure is substantially less than that experienced during a barium enema. With shorter data acquisition and analysis times resulting in lower costs for this technology, it is likely that virtual colonoscopy will replace some of the techniques currently used for screening for CRC.

Magnetic resonance colonography

Recent work in Europe has sought to evaluate the utility of magnetic resonance colonography [13]. The preparation of the patient for this procedure involves instillation of water and a gadolinium based contrast agent into the colon. As for spiral CT virtual colonoscopy a single breath hold data acquisition sequence is used, although it may be repeated several times with the patient in different positions to help to determine the presence of residual fecal material in the colon. It appears that adenomatous lesions are enhanced by the gadolinium, thus further helping diagnostic specificity of this technique. Further data are required to demonstrate any clinical benefits over the technique of virtual endoscopy using spiral CT.

Improvements in mucosal definition

Optical coherence tomography with micron scale imaging [14] and endoscopic laser-induced fluorescence spectroscopy [15] are being utilized in experimental protocols to aid detection of dysplastic lesions in the upper and lower gastrointestinal tract. Likewise, photodynamic diagnosis is being utilized for the detection of dysplasia and cancer in the esophagus and stomach [16, 17].

Although these methods currently rely on passage of an endoscopic instrument into the lumen of the GIT, it is conceivable that the technology underlying these techniques may be harnessed in a virtual reality system to provide more accurate non-invasive screening tools.

Speculative modalities

A number of novel modalities may well be applied to technologies currently available to enhance the prospects of non-invasive screening techniques.

Preliminary studies of monoclonal antibody-labelled gadolinium to selectively detect colonic adenomas in rats have thus far been unsuccessful, but it is likely that approaches aimed at targeting lesions prior to imaging will increase diagnostic utility of non-invasive techniques in the future.

Harmonic ultrasound may improve resolution of hepatic lesions allowing earlier detection and treatment of hepatocellular carcinoma [18].

Space age robotics and microcomputers may in the not too distant future result in the availability of ingestable video chips with the potential to treat lesions that are detected during their passage through the colon.

Summary and conclusions

Simple, cheap, non-invasive methods of screening for hepatobiliary, pancreatic and GI malignancies are still some way off, and there is no immediate likelihood of endoscopy being superseded by radiological techniques in the immediate future. However, it is likely that the advances in imaging of the colon that are occurring today will result in similar changes that have occurred in the practice of ERCP. Diagnostic colonoscopy may well become a thing of the past and it will become increasingly important for gastroenterologists to receive adequate training in therapeutic endoscopy. This will require revision of training guidelines and requirements for continuing education, but will ensure that the next generation of gastroenterologists is equipped to deal with the lesions detected by highly sophisticated imaging systems and molecular biological techniques.

At present we should focus on adequately utilizing currently available techniques such as chromoendoscopy (Barrett's and gastric carcinoma), ultrasound (hepatoma), endoscopic ultrasound (rectal carcinoma) and colonoscopy.

Well-designed and adequately controlled trials must be performed to assess outcomes of any screeing program utilizing new technology, and our excitement at the prospects provided by virtual reality images must be tempered by hard clinical data.

References

1. Winawer SJ, Zauber AG, Gerdes H, O'Brien MJ, Gottlieb LS, Sternberg SS, Bond JH, Waye JD, Schapiro M, Panish JF, *et al. DDW* 1994. Abstract.
2. Hix WR, Wilson WR. Toluidine Blue Staining of the Esophagus: A useful adjunct in the panendoscopic evaluation of patients with squamous cell carcinoma of the head and neck. *Arch Otolaryngol, Head and Neck Surg* 1987; 1 (13): 864-5.
3. Seitz JF, Monges G, Navarro P, Giovannini M, Gauthier A. Endoscopic detection of dysplasia and early esophageal cancer: results of a prospective study of toluidine blue vital staining in 100 tobacco and alcohol users. *Gastroenterol. Clin Biol* 1990; 14: 15-21.
4. Nabeya K, Hanaoka T, Onozawa K, Nyumura T, Kaku. Early diagnosis of esophageal cancer. *Hepato-gastroenterology* 1990; 37: 368-70.
5. Misumi A, Harada K, Murakami A, Arima K, Kondo H, Akagi M, Yagi Y, Ikeda T, Baba K, Kobori Y, Matsukane H. Role of Lugol dye endoscopy in diagnosis of early esophageal cancer. *Endoscopy* 1990; 22: 12-6.
6. Chisolm EM, Williams SR, Leung JW, Chung SC, Van Hasselt CA, Li AK. Lugol's iodine dye-enhanced endoscopy in patients with cancer of the oesophagus and head and neck. *Eur J Surg Oncol* 1992; 16: 550-2.
7. Shiozaki H, Tahara H, Kobayashi K, Yano H, Tamura S, Imamoto H, Yano T, Oku K, Miyata M, Nishiyama K, Kubo K, Mori T. Endoscopic screening of early esophageal cancer with the lugol dye method in patients with head and neck cancers. *Cancer* 1990; 66: 2068-71.
8. Ina H, Shibuya H, Ohashi I, Kitagawa M. The frequency of a concomitant early esophageal cancer in male patients with oral and oropharyngeal cancer. *Cancer* 1994; 73: 2038-41.
9. Lightdale CJ. Endoscopy in premalignant conditions of the esophagus. *Gastrointest Endosc* 1984; 30: 308-10.
10. Iishi H, Tatsuta M, Okuda S. Diagnosis of simultaneous multiple gastric cancers by the endoscopic congo red-methylene blue test. *Endoscopy* 1988; 20: 78-82.
11. Fennerty MB, Sampliner RE, McGee DL, Hixson LJ, Garewal HS. Intestinal metaplasia of the stomach: identification by a selective mucosal staining technique. *Gastrointest Endosc* 1992; 38: 696-8.
12. Tatsuta M, Iishi H, Ichii M, Noguchi S, Okuda S, Taniguchi H. Chromoendoscopic observations on extension and development of fundal gastritis and intestinal metaplasia. *Gastroenterology* 1985; 88: 70-4.
13. Chung JB, Seo JH, Kim MJ, Kang JK, Park IS. Magnetic Resonance Cholangiopancreatography in the diagnosis of extrahepatic bile duct cancer: comparison with endoscopic retrograde cholangiopancreatography. *DDW* 1998. Abstract 246.
14. Vining DJ, Gelfand DW. Non-invasive colonoscopy using helical CT scanning, 3D reconstruction, and virtual reality. Presented at the Society of Gastrointestinal Radiologists Annual Meeting, Maui, HT, Feb, 1994.
15. Vining D, Ge Y, Ahn D, Stelts D, Pineau B. Enhanced virtual colonoscopy system employing automatic detection of colonic polyps. *DDW* 1998.
16. Luboldt W, Bauerfeind P, Steiner P, Fried M, Krestin GP, Debatin JF. Preliminary assessment of three-dimensional magnetic resonance imaging for various colonic disorders. *Lancet* 1997; 349: 1288-91.
17. Brezinski ME, Pitris C, Boppart SA, Fujimoto JG. Micron scale imaging of the gastrointestinal tract with optical coherence tomography. *DDW* 1998. Abstract 574.
18. Brand S, Ochsenkuhn T, Stepp H, Baumgartner R, Weinzierl M, Holl J, V. Ritter C, Paumgartner G, Sackmann M. Detection of low grade colonic dysplasia by light-induced fluorescence endoscopy. *DDW* 1998. Abstract 622.

19. Murata Y, Matsui H, Hirano K, Yanaka A, Nakahara A, Muto H. Gastric cancer areas can be diagnosed by porphyrin fluorescence with a simultaneous endoscopic fluorescence analyzing system at photodynamic therapy. *DDW* 1998. Abstract 635.
20. Gossner L, Stepp H, Sroka R, May A, Stolte M, Ell C. Photodynamic diagnosis of high grade dysplasia and early cancer of the upper GI-tract using 5-aminolaevulinnic (ALA). *DDW* 1998. Abstract 3384.
21. Hayakawa S, Goto H, Hirooka Y, Itoh A, Watanabe Y, Ishiguro Y, Kojima S, Hashimoto S, Hayakawa T, Naitoh Y, Burns PN, Powers JE. A new ultrasound imaging method in the abdominal area: harmonic imaging without an enhancing agent. *DDW* 1998. Abstract 234.

Pharmacology
in hepatology and gastroenterology
in the next Millenium

What is to be expected in acid related disorders: acid control and *Helicobacter pylori*

G. Sachs[1], J.M. Shin[1], M. Besançon[1], N. Lambrecht[1], D. Scott[1], D. Weeks[1], D. Melle[1], K. Melchers[2]

[1] *UCLA and Wadsworth VA Hospital, Los Angeles Ca, USA;* [2] *Byk Gulden, Konstanz, Germany*

There has been a major revolution in the understanding and treatment of ulcer disease in the last quarter of this century. The drivers of this late-breaking revolution were several: understanding of the regulation of acid secretion and its mechanism, improved visualization of the lesions using flexible endoscopes, improved surgical approaches, more sophisticated pharmaceutical research and the discovery of *H. pylori* and its implication in ulcer disease to name a few.

We are still arguing about the personality of *H. pylori*. Is it always a pathogen? Is it merely a commensal on occasion, hindering rather than helping to initiate disease? The early part of the century should provide an answer to this conundrum. Treatment of acid related disease has been successful, treatment of gastric or esophageal malignancies is not. Robotic surgery coupled with imaging technology may bring a level of precision enabling levels of curative extirpation impossible today.

We await the complete human genome, with its more than 100,000 genes. From this we will learn about, perhaps more rapidly than we can understand, the changes in gene expression in different cell types that orchestrate growth and differentiation and that diagnose the presence or the prediction of one or more of life's many ills. A crowd, a host of new therapeutic targets will be provided. Among them, will there be novel lower esophageal sphincter receptors, host predictors of *H. pylori* pathogenicity or tumorogenicity?

In this brief review, we shall try to cover two areas, that of the possible future of acid control and of *H. pylori* eradication, visiting the "past", the present and the future, in terms of possible therapies.

The "past"

Although much remains to be discovered in this area, especially in neural regulation, the past is used since it is unlikely that therapies targeted against receptors will provide significant additional benefit as compared to currently available therapy.

Acid control

The first three quarters of this century were devoted to defining mechanisms of regulation of acid secretion and to arguments as to the nature of acid secretion itself, a redox pump such as exists in mitochondria or an ATP based proton transporter. Many of these questions appear to have been resolved but some are still mysterious.

Receptors regulating gastric acid secretion
Mechanisms of stimulation of acid secretion

A triumvirate of cells, the ECL cell, the G cell and the D cell interact to regulate the function of the parietal cell. Endocrine, paracrine and neurocrine mediators of regulation of these cells and the parietal cell have been described.

- Cholinergic mediation

That atropine inhibited acid secretion had been known, at least indirectly, for many centuries, but with the discovery of acetylcholine and thence muscarinic and nicotinic mechanisms, the effect of atropine could be ascribed to interference with muscarinic stimulation of acid secretion. With novel chemicals and cloning technologies, five separate muscarinic receptors were discovered. Of this, the M1, 3 and 5 subtypes were found to be activating and the others inhibitory. Two relatively selective M1 antagonists, pirenzepine and telenzepine, were found to be inhibitors of acid secretion, although still not free of side effects.

The gastric parietal cell, the source of acid secretion, was found, pharmacologically and by RT-PCR to have a M3 receptor, suggesting that the M1 receptors responsible for the efficacy of inhibition of acid secretion by pirenzepine are located upstream in the stimulatory pathway of acid secretion. Various possibilities as to the location are the ECL cell, the G cell or within the neurons of the myenteric plexus. In the former, these receptors mediate peripheral regulation of acid secretion, in the latter the M1 receptors would be involved in mediation of the central regulation of acid secretion.

In recent years, it has been possible to isolate and study functional responses in purified ECL cells and in functionally defined G and D cells. Surprisingly, only about 20% of the ECL cells respond to carbachol, whereas all respond to gastrin. Whether this is due to damage to the M receptor on the ECL cell during isolation, or whether this is due to only a sub-population of ECL cells is not clear, but confocal microscopy of isolated gastric glands may provide the answer to this problem.

- Gastrin

The role of this hormone in stimulation of acid secretion has had a checkered history since its controversial discovery by Edkins at the beginning of the century. Its re-establishment as a central player in endocrine regulation of acid was due to the efforts of Komarov. The sequencing of gastrin by Tracy and Gregory and the development of radio-immunoassay by Yalow and Berson gave fresh impetus to investigations of the role of gastrin in acid secretion. The development of H2 receptor antagonists and isolated rabbit gastric glands showed that the effect of gastrin on acid secretion was indirect probably mediated by histamine. Histamine release from isolated purified ECL cells stimulated by calcium signals resulting from gastrin binding to a CCK-B receptor provided a firm experimental basis for the major effect of gastrin on gastric acid secretion.

The undoubted presence of a CCK-B receptor on the parietal cell raises the issue as to its function. Clearly, this receptor is linked to calcium signaling, as is the M3 receptor. The M3 receptor can induce an acid secretory response in parietal cells in the face of H2 antagonists whereas gastrin cannot. One hypothesis, with some experimental support, is that elevation of cAMP must accompany gastrin binding to the CCK-B receptor for the calcium signal to be observed.

- Histamine

The synthesis and development of H2 receptor antagonists in the 1970's heralded a new era not only in the pharmacology of acid secretion but also in the treatment of acid related diseases. The idea of H2 receptors as compared to the H1 receptors depended on the recognition that H1 receptor antagonists were relatively ineffective at blocking acid secretion. With the introduction of cimetidine, acid related disorders became amenable to rational drug therapy and vastly expanded treatment of upper GI distress ensued and several antagonists were marketed. The pharmacology of these antagonists established the major role of histamine as a paracrine mediator of acid secretion.

There were limitations, however, on their clinical efficacy. For example, elevation of day time pH was rather poor, hence treatment of reflux esophagitis was relatively poor. Their usefulness in combination with antibiotics for eradication of *H. pylori* was very limited. Further they suffer from epiphenomena such as tolerance and acid rebound. For this reason, proton pump inhibitors now seem to dominate the prescription market.

The histamine 2 receptor has been cloned and mutagenesis studies have defined an amine binding pocket in the 3rd and 5th transmembrane segments, as for other amine responsive receptors.

- Neural mediation

When it was shown that carbachol was a relatively ineffective stimulant of the isolated ECL cell, this raised the issue of the neural mediator that stimulated acid secretion. Pituitary Adenylate Cyclase Activating Peptide (PACAP) was found to be an effective stimulant of ECL cell calcium signaling and histamine release as well as of ECL cell growth. When injected along with neutralizing somatostatin antibody, PACAP produced stimulation of gastric acid secretion. It seems then that PACAP is a candidate as a neural mediator of centrally activated acid secretion given that it is found in nerves of the stomach.

Mechanisms of inhibition of gastric acid secretion
- Somatostatin

This peptide is contained within antral and fundic D cells. The former communicate with the antral gland lumen and are thought to release somatostatin as a function of acidification of the lumen. The peptide is relatively short lived and probably acts locally to inhibit gastrin release from the G cell. The D cells have receptors for both CCK-A and CCK-B as well as inhibitory muscarinic receptors. Somatostatin also inhibits ECL cell function at a type 2 subtype of somatostatin receptor. It would seem to be the major peripheral down regulator of gastric acid secretion. Somatostatin analogs have been synthesized that have proved useful in localizing gastrinomas but not for inhibition of gastric acid secretion.

- Galanin

This neuropeptide is found in gastric nerves and is able to inhibit isolated ECL cell function. It therefore is a candidate for neural mediation of central inhibition of gastric acid secretion. It inhibits histamine release and calcium signaling and Gal R1 receptors are responsible for the effect based on RT-PCR.

A model that ensues for regulation of acid secretion at the level of the ECL cell considers this cell as the major regulator of parietal cell function, the point of intersection of neural and endocrine/paracrine regulation of acid secretion *(figure 1)*.

Pathogenesis of ulcer disease
The re-discovery of *H. pylori* in association with peptic ulcers and its establishment as a major contributory factor to the causation of this disease was a milestone in understanding of duodenal and gastric ulcer generation. It was realized as more epidemiology was determined that only a fraction of the individuals infected actually contracted disease and further that infection contributed little to non-ulcer dyspepsia. This dilemma resembles the "no acid no ulcer" concept where it was recognized that only a few people with acid secretion had peptic ulcers. Now that the organism was established as implicated, much effort has been expended trying to relate characteristics of the organism to its pathogenicity. Products of the pathogenicity island, with cag A as a marker, vac A or ice as cytotoxins may be implicated, but it is more complicated than an all or none property of the organism. Still we have to invoke unknown properties of the patient as contributing to the disease. Also early in the history of the organism, the importance of its urease activity as a neutralizing factor for gastric acidity was recognized, although most emphasis was placed on the surface urease of the bacterium as enabling its gastric survival and colonization. Further epidemiological studies pointed to the phenomenon of gastric fundic atrophy caused

by fundic infestation as a pre-cancerous condition leading to the classification of the organism as a class I carcinogen. Elimination of this organism became an international priority.

As the concept of *H. pylori* became more established, essentially a trial and error approach was taken to eradication of the organism with a view to curing ulcer disease. Only recently has there been a systematic investigation in a sufficiently large population of patients with the usual criteria for clinical trials determining the efficacies of a variety of triple therapies on a twice a day regimen. It appears that any therapy using amoxicillin and clarithromycin (or perhaps metronidazole) in combination with a proton pump inhibitor generates essentially equivalent data with between 80 and 90% success.

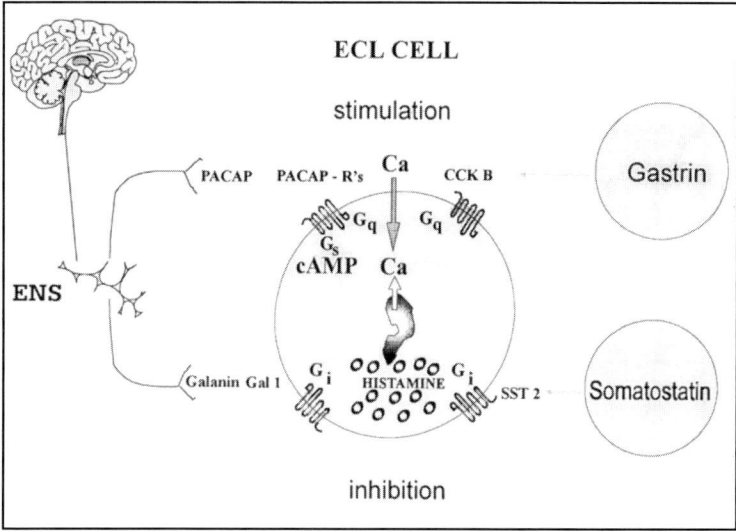

Figure 1. A model of regulation of ECL cell function by the enteric nervous system (ENS) and the gastric endocrine system.

The "present"

Acid control

The recognition that the final step of acid secretion was a H/K exchange P type ATPase made this a natural target for anti ulcer drugs. The hope was also that inhibition of this pump would reduce the acid load on the gastric mucosa and the duodenum sufficiently so as to optimize healing and further, reduce the refluxed acid load on the esophageal epithelium so as to improve the outcome for treatment of reflux esophagitis.

The gastric acid pump is an alpha-beta heterodimer. The alpha subunit is the catalytic component of the enzyme which converts the energy of ATP breakdown into outward transport of H and inward transport of K. The beta subunit is essential for assembly of the enzyme, membrane targeting and for stabilizing the necessary conformation. The linear amino acid sequence of the two subunits of the pump are known. The catalytic subunit has ten transmembrane segments, the beta subunit only one. The arrangement of the alpha and beta subunits has been worked out in part, but we are far from a detailed 3 dimensional structure of the pump. From mutagenesis and binding studies it appears that the 5th and 6th transmembrane segments might be important in ion transport by this and other mammalian P type ATPases and would be a target for inhibitors of the enzyme *(figure 2)*.

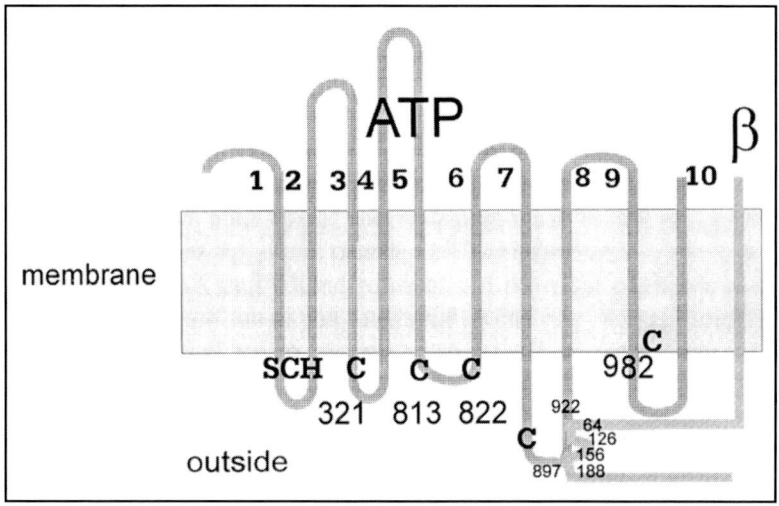

Figure 2. The membrane segments of the H,K ATPase illustrating the cysteines on the luminal surface and the regions of interaction between the alpha and beta subunits.

Omeprazole, the first of the proton pump inhibitors (PPI's), was synthesized in 1979 and launched in 1988. Other proton pump inhibitors have also been developed, lansoprazole, pantoprazole and rabeprazole. The mechanism of these is in principle very similar. They are all protonatable weak bases, with a pK_a of 4.0 with rabeprazole at 4.9. As a function of this pK_a these compounds accumulate in acidic spaces with a pH less than the pK_a. The only acidic space known in the human body with a $pH_i < 4.0$ is the acidic space of the secreting parietal cell. Following this stimulation dependent accumulation, the compounds undergo an acid catalyzed rearrangement to generate a thiophilic compound, a sulfenamide in aqueous solutions as illustrated in *figure 3*.

The reactive thiophile binds covalently to the enzyme, and the stable covalent bond critical for inhibition by omeprazole is at cys 813. Inhibition by the other PPI's also involves this cysteine, but other cysteines may also react covalently with the inhibitors. The PPI's are therefore prodrugs requiring gastric acid secretion for their efficacy. The compounds differ in their rate of acid activation where rabeprazole > omeprazole = lansoprazole > pantoprazole. This difference does not appear to have any clinical consequence as yet but the mechanism of action has interesting pharmacological implications.

Not all parietal cells are active at any one time, and not all parietal cells are equally active. The cells in the neck region are new cells, those deeper in the gland are older cells which also express different membrane transporters, such as the $NaKCl_2$ cotransporter. The effective plasma half-life of the PPI's appears to be about 60-90 minutes and inhibition of acid secretion is related to area under the curve (AUC) rather than to peak height. The inhibition of the pump will occur essentially only during the time that the drug is present at effective concentrations in the blood provided that the pump is also actively secreting acid. It is therefore important to administer the drugs along with or prior to food and in the absence of other means of inhibition of acid secretion.

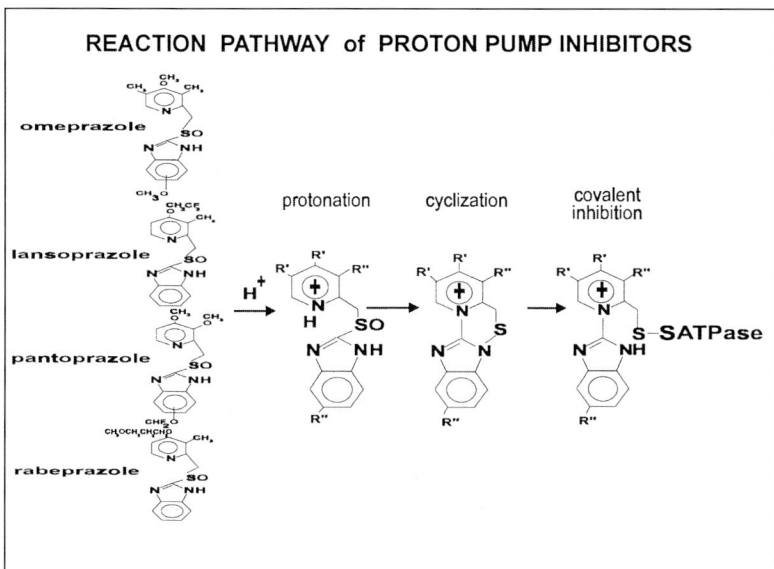

Figure 3. The chemistry of the PPI's.

The first dose will inhibit secretion immediately but given that a fraction of the pumps are inactive, acid secretion will recommence after the drug has disappeared from plasma. The pumps that were active are inhibited covalently so by the time the next dose is given, these pumps have largely remained inhibited but some of pumps that were previously inactive will now be active and be inhibited by the next dose. The pump is also constantly synthesized and in the rat the $t_{1/2}$ of turnover is about 50 hrs. If one assumes that at time of administration 75% of pumps are inhibitable, then steady state inhibition is reached after about three days. pH metric analysis will show inhibition of day time acidity but weaker effects at night since the pumps synthesized during the day will never have seen drug. Furthermore, in the absence of food, given a constant output of 160 mM H^+ by any active pump, there will be periods of acidity where intragastric pH falls to below 2.0.

Notwithstanding these theoretical drawbacks, all the PPI's have been shown to be superior to H2 receptor antagonists in treatment of peptic ulcers, reflux disease and synergism with antibiotics for eradication of *H. pylori*.

Pathogenesis of ulcer disease

Knowledge has begun to accumulate about the specific genetic constitution of *H. pylori* since its full genome has been sequenced. Of probable special interest are the proteins known to be membrane expressed since these must form a line of defense for the organism against gastric acidity. Some of these may be unique to the organism and hence form selective targets for eradication *(figure 4)*.

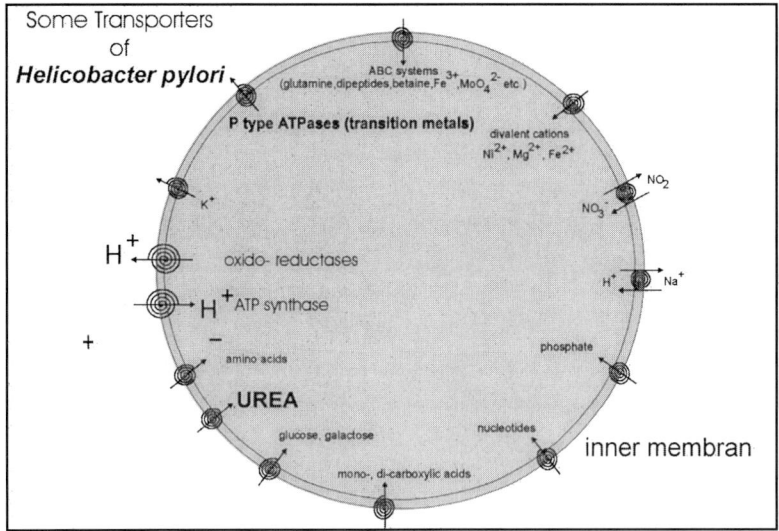

Figure 4. The membrane transporters identified in the genome of *H. pylori*.

More is now understood about the mechanisms surrounding gastric colonization by the organism. It is a Gram negative neutralophile that has adapted to the gastric environment particularly because of its production of large quantities of urease, which by hydrolyzing urea, produces ammonia to neutralize acidity. Studies on the survival of the organism *in vitro* have shown that it can only survive between pH 4.0 and 8.0 in the absence of urea and that it grows between pH 6.0 and 8.0. In the presence of urea it can survive a medium pH of 2.0 since urease activity rapidly elevates medium pH. However also in the presence of urea it does not survive at a pH of 8.0 since alkalinization of the medium takes place. At a pH of less than 2.0 the urease activity is not able to maintain life.

In terms of survival or growth, it is vital for the organism to maintain the sum of the pH gradient and the potential difference across its inner membrane constant to allow for ATP and protein synthesis. It therefore has developed a mechanism for regulating its internal urease activity so that the periplasmic pH is kept at 6.2 and transmembrane potential at about – 100 mV allowing for survival and growth in gastric acidity without having to neutralize gastric acid outside *(figure 5)*.

In accordance with the expectation for survival, urease negative mutants do not colonize any animal model. The urease gene cluster, often called the urease operon, consists of ure A and B, the urease proteins, and ure I, E,F,G and H. The specific function of these genes is not known.

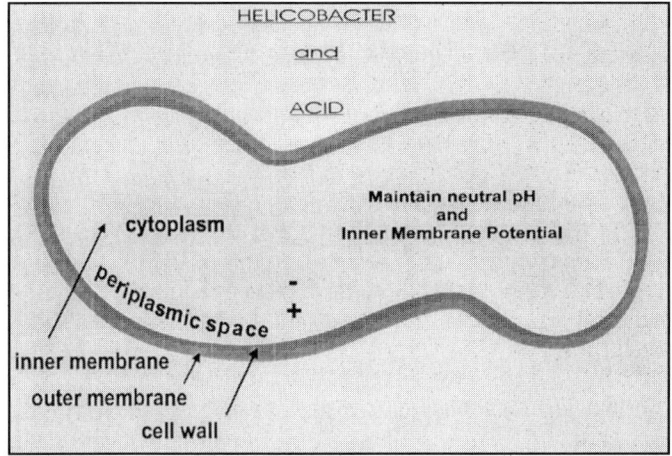

Figure 5. The elementary structure of *H. pylori* showing the boundaries of the periplasmic space and the necessity for maintenance of pH gradient and inner membrane potential.

The "future"

It is rash to predict what is going to happen in the field of acid related disorders. Imagine writing this in 1970, before the first H2 receptor antagonist had been devised, or in 1977 before the first proton pump inhibitor had had its antisecretory mechanism deduced or even 1982, before *H. pylori* fell on a skeptical group of acidophobes. Nevertheless we shall try to make some short sighted predictions.

Acid control

The PPI's are excellent drugs for the control of acid secretion and suspicions as to their safety are fading. In many instances they are regarded as reserve, overly effective drugs. The phrase often used is "cannonballs shooting sparrows". Hunting in many places in the world is not averse to this unequal match. Probably these drugs will become universally prescribed as first line therapy if no other issues arise and as they become cheaper with the advent of generic forms of the medication. They are however not perfect in that they do not ablate acid secretion at any time, nor do they act very rapidly.

Their mechanism on the pump itself may be more complicated than once thought. Mutagenesis studies seem to suggest that there is initially a reversible binding in the region of cys # 822 followed by covalent binding to cys 813. Apparently both cysteines are necessary for inhibition by omeprazole. Whether this explains the puzzlingly rapid restoration of ATPase activity and acid secretion in the rat following treatment by omeprazole is not clear as yet. Obviously this is a field for transgenic analysis.

A second type of drug is being developed for inhibition of the proton pump, based on the structure of SCH 28080, a 1,2 [α] imidazo-pyridine. This class of drug is K competitive and does not bind to the pump covalently and is independent of the functional status of the pump. These acid pump antagonists, APA's, if proven to be safe and effective, will rapidly elevate intragastric pH to neutrality and act as therapeutic antacids. They are acid stable not requiring special formulation to survive gastric acidity and even begin their absorption across the gastric wall.

In order to understand their mechanism of action, their sites of binding will have to be defined as related to a more realistic image of the H,K ATPase requiring higher and higher 3 dimensional resolution, by diffraction of 2D or 3D crystals and dedicated site directed mutagenesis. If these drugs reach the market it will be interesting to see whether their more rapid effect and non-covalent binding will impinge on a market dominated by PPI's.

What about reflux disease? Exposure of the esophagus to acidity greater than pH 3.0 results in pain and/or erosion. Do we need even better acid control than that offered by PPI's? Should these be reformulated to give rapid and continuous suppression so that the pH never falls to less than 4.0? Or will APA's be able to provide the degree of acid suppression to give full symptom relief in ambulatory reflux and also given at night deal with night time reflux and laryngitis?

Pathogenesis of ulcer disease

Perhaps the more innovative prospect is the likely explosion in the understanding of the biology of *H. pylori* resulting in definition of its mechanism of epithelial damage, immunocyte recruitment and genes that form novel therapeutic targets.

For example, the regulation of internal urease activity depends on expression of ure I, a gene in the urease cluster. This is an integral membrane protein, homologous to genes in the amidase operon of other organisms. Its role may well be that of urea transport with activation below 6.2. This would be an interesting eradication target if the organism is subjected to a pH < 4.0 since this is when urease activity is essential and free urease is inactive at this pH.

Many believe that the gastric surface pH is significantly higher than luminal pH, for example being close to neutrality when luminal pH is > 2.0. Recent work with the confocal microscope suggests that the finding of this pH gradient may be an artefact of microelectrode measurements. Certainly if this were the case, why would *H. pylori* require highly effective acid adaptive mechanisms and why would other neutralophiles not be found in the stomach? Is there more to the gastric barrier than simple impermeability of the apical membranes of the gastric epithelial cells? Perhaps not.

Eradication will then move away from the use of general antibiotics. This might also open the door to a more general approach to eradication, not just for symptomatic patients. This might also serve as an introduction for vaccination against the organism particularly in underdeveloped countries where availability of new drugs and compliance is an issue.

The effects of the bacterial infection on acid secretion and epithelial integrity are beginning to be understood. Perhaps as the human genome and the genes displayed in normal and abnormal epithelium are defined, understanding of the origins of ulcer disease will expand. Will there be substantiation of the organism as largely a commensal and an occasional pathogen? Will ulcer therapy begin to target the abnormal genes in the human epithelium? A crystal ball has insufficient focus to answer these questions.

Bibliography

- Black JW, Duncan WAM, Durant CJ, Ganellin CR, Parsons ME. Definition and antagonism of histamine H2 receptors. *Nature* 1972; 236: 385.
- Feldman M, Burton ME. Histamine H2 receptor antagonists. *N Engl J Med* 1990; 323: 1672.
- Feldman M. Inhibition of gastric acid secretion by selective and nonselective anticholinergics. *Gastroenterology* 1984; 86: 361.
- Kopin AS, Lee YM, McBride EW, Miller LJ, Lu M, Lin HY, Kolakowski LF, Jr., Beinborn M. Expression cloning and characterization of the canine parietal cell gastrin receptor. *Proc Natl Acad Sci USA* 1992; 89: 3605-9.
- Gantz I, Schaeffer M, DelValle J, Logsdon C, Campbell V, Uhler M, Yamada T. Molecular cloning of a gene encoding the histamine H2-receptor. *Proc Natl Acad Sci USA* 1991; 488: 429.
- Warren JR, Marshall B. Unidentified curved bacilli on gastric epithelium in active chronic gastritis. *Lancet* 1983; i: 1273-5.
- Lind T, Veldhuyzen van Zanten S, Unge P, et al. Eradication of *Helicobacter pylori* using one-week triple therapies combining omeprazole with two antimicrobials the MACH I Study. *Helicobacter* 1996; 1: 138-44.
- Misiewicz JJ, Harris AW, Bardhan KD, et al. One week triple therapy for *Helicobacter pylori*: a multicentre comparative study. Lansoprazole Helicobacter Study Group. *Gut* 1997; 41: 735-9.
- Parsonnet J, Friedman GD, Vandersteed DP, et al. H. pylori infection and the risk of gastric cancer. *N Engl J Med* 1991; 325: 1131.
- Rauws EA, Tytgat GN. Cure of duodenal ulcer associated with eradication of *Helicobacter pylori*. *Eur J Gastroenterol Hepatol* 1990; 6: 773-7.
- Graham DY. *Campylobacter pylori* and peptic ulcer disease. *Gastroenterology* 1989; 96: 615-25.
- Axon ATR. Eradication of *Helicobacter pylori*. *Scand J Gastroenterol* 1996; 31: 47-53.
- Brandstrom A, Lindberg P, Bergman NA, Alminger T, Ankner K, Junggren U, Lamm B, Nordberg P, Erickson M, Grundevik I, Hagin I, Hoffmann KJ, Johansson S, Larsson S, Lofberg I, Ohlson K, Persson B, Skönberg I, Tekenbergs-Hjelte L. Chemical Reactions of Omeprazole and Omeprazole Analogues. I. A Survey of the Chemical Transformations of Omeprazole and its Analogues. *Acta Chem Scand* 1989; 43: 536-611.

- Besancon M, Simon A, Sachs G, Shin JM. Sites of Reaction of the Gastric H,K-ATPase with Extracytoplasmic Thiol Reagents. *J Biol Chem* 1997; 272: 22438-46.
- Mobley HLT, Island MD, Hausinger RP. Molecular biology of microbial ureases. *Microbiol Rev* 1995; 59: 451-80.
- Meyer-Rosberg K, Scott DR, Rex D, Melchers K, Sachs G. The effect of the environmental pH on the proton motive force of *Helicobacter pylori*. *Gastroenterology* 1996; 111: 886-900.
- Clyne M, Labigne A, Drumm B. *Helicobacter pylori* requires an acidic environment to survive in the presence of urea. *Infect Immun* 1995; 63: 1669-73.
- Sanders MJ, Ayalon A, Roll M, Soll AH. The apical surface of canine chief cell monolayers resists H^+ back-diffusion. *Nature* 1985; 313: 52-3.
- Verdu EF, Armstrong D, Idstrom JP, Labenz J, Stolte M, Dorta G, Borsch G, Blum AL. Effect of curing *Helicobacter pylori* infection on intragastric pH during treatment with omeprazole. *Gut* 1995; 37: 743-8.
- Walsh JH, Peterson WL. The treatment of *Helicobacter pylori* infection in the management of peptic ulcer disease. *N Engl J Med* 1995; 333: 984-91.
- Kuipers EJ, Klinkenberg-Knol EC, Vandenbroucke-Grauls CM, Appelmelk BJ, Schenk BE, Meuwissen SG. Role of *Helicobacter pylori* in the pathogenesis of atrophic gastritis. *Scand J Gastroenterol* 1997; suppl. 223: 28-34.
- Labenz J, Tillenburg B, Peitz U, Idstrom JP, Verdu E, Stolte M, Borsch G, Blum A. *Helicobacter pylori* augments the pH-increasing effect of omeprazole in patients with duodenal ulcer. *Gastroenterology* 1996; 110: 725-32.
- Lee A, Dixon MF, Danon SJ, Kuipers E, Megraud F, Larsson H, Mellgard B. Local acid production and *Helicobacter pylori*: a unifying hypothesis of gastroduodenal disease. *Eur J Gastroenterol Hepatol* 1995; 7: 461-5.
- McGowan CC, Cover TL, Blaser MJ. *Helicobacter pylori* and gastric acid: biological and therapeutic implications. *Gastroenterology* 1996; 110: 926-38.
- Sachs G, Shin JM, Briving C, Wallmark B, Hersey S. Pharmacology of gastric H,K ATPase. *Ann Rev Pharm Toxic* 1995; 35: 277-305.
- Swarts HG, Klaassen CH, de Boer M, Fransen JA, De Pont JJ. Role of negatively charged residues in the fifth and sixth transmembrane domains of the catalytic subunit of gastric H+,K+-ATPase. *J Biol Chem* 1996; 271: 29764-72.
- Larsson H, Carlsson E, Mattsson H. Plasma gastrin in gastric enterochromaffin-like cell activation and proliferation: studies with omeprazole and ranitidine in intact and antrectomized rats. *Gastroenterology* 1986; 90: 391-9.
- Scott DR, Weeks D, Hong C, Postius S, Melchers K, Sachs G. The role of internal urease in acid resistance of *Helicobacter pylori*. *Gastroenterology* 1998; 114: 58-70.

Can cholesterol gallstones be prevented?

M.C. Carey

Brigham and Women's Hospital/Harvard Medical School,
Boston, USA

An unequivocal "yes" can be given to the title question, since fundamental aspects of cholesterol gallstone disease have reached an advanced stage of maturity. This is particularly so with respect to basic knowledge of its physical-chemical etiology and pathogenesis; however, much less is known concerning the metabolic/molecular basis of cholesterol gallstones, particularly their genetic origin. Cholesterol gallstones are endemic in Westernized countries and cause much morbidity and mortality, particularly since the leading treatment option is cholecystectomy, a major surgical procedure. Strategies to prevent any common worldwide disease are meritorious, but one must appreciate the more practical driving forces to do so. Gallstone disease today is the most expensive digestive disease. In the United States of America, it has been has been estimated that the disease costs $8 billion a year, or 1.5% of total health care costs.

Details of why prevention is desirable

The enormous cost and suffering caused by gallstone disease includes i) morbidity, 20% of patients with pain, also anxiety, absenteeism; ii) complications in 1-5% (cholecystitis, choledocholithiasis, cholangitis, pancreatitis, gallbladder cancer); iii) surgical complications in 3-5% (bile leaks, "lost" stones, pancreatitis, bile duct/bowel injury, ERCP required in 10% of laparoscopic cholecystectomies, "lap choly"); iv) mortality, principally from surgery, estimated at 3,000/yr in the USA; moreover; v) in 5-15% of patients, cholecystectomy is misdirected in that the abdominal pain had another cause that was unrelated to gallstones, and therefore persists; vi) chronic diarrhea following surgery in 1-5% of patients; some of these patients require therapy with bile salt sequestrants for life.

Current therapies for cholesterol gallstone patients

– The recommended option for gallstone patients with no symptoms or non-specific dyspepsia, or equivocal biliary pain is reassurance and watchful waiting. Biliary pain is not a "colic", always lasts more than thirty minutes and in 80% of sufferers is nocturnal, occurring within two hours of retiring.

– Symptomatic gallstone patients require intervention, and this is usually surgery, "lap choly" in 90%, conventional or open cholecystectomy in 10%.

– Dissolution with oral bile acids, ursodeoxycholic acid, UCDA (ursodiol), or chenodoxycholic acid, CDCA (chenodiol), or a combination of both, gives satisfactory results in only 10% or less and is best suited for patients with floating stones 5-7 mm in maximal diameter.

– Extracorporeal shock-wave lithotripsy (ESWL) found a niche in several European and Asian centers, but enthusiasm was never high with gallstone patients or their physicians in the USA ESWL is suitable only for selected patients, particularly those with large single stones and normal gallbladder function.

– ESWL may be combined with oral dissolution of stone fragments, but if fragmentation is sufficiently fine and the gallbladder contracts appropriately, bile acid therapy is not required.

– Contact dissolution with a cholesterol-dissolving organic solvent *via* a transhepatic or percutaneous catheter in the gallbladder. This is now considered a highly invasive procedure that is not without risk, and therefore probably should be considered experimental only. Apart from surgery, all treatment modalities are associated with the risk of stones recurring, which is the case with 70% of patients within 5-10 years.

Cholesterol gallstone formation: key concepts

Three principal abnormalities are essential for cholesterol gallstone formation.

– A solubility defect: bile must be supersaturated with cholesterol and this is caused by secretion of more cholesterol molecules from the liver into bile than can be solubilized by bile salts and lecithins in the solubilizing particles, which are simple plus mixed micelles. It is agreed generally that "supersaturated bile" is a misnomer and that bile with excess cholesterol contains, in addition to micelles, unilamellar phospholipid-cholesterol vesicles. By definition, therefore, lithogenic bile is actually a two-phase system.

– A residence time defect: the gallbladder in cholesterol gallstone disease is "large, lax and lazy". In addition to a large fasting volume, which empties sluggishly and incompletely, there is a large residual volume. Lipid concentration dynamics are also important, in that speed and extent of dehydration of hepatic bile is critical for facilitating solid crystallization on a physiological time-scale.

– A kinetic defect, that is, the speed with which the metastable state relaxes into the equilibrium or near-equilibrium state, which is defined in the well known "bile" phase diagram. Nucleation in bile is always heterogeneous, that is, requires a nucleating agent to allow solid crystals to form on a matrix, which is usually mucin gel. Crystal growth is accelerated by a number of factors, including the degree of supersaturation as codified in the Cholesterol Saturation Index (CSI) and the calcium content of bile. There are other promoters and possibly inhibitors of both nucleation and crystallization in bile, but the true pathophysiological role of these is controversial. Hypersecretion of cholesterol by the liver can affect many secondary defects such as prolonging gallbladder residence time. Further, rapid nucleation may be a result of chemical injury to the gallbladder by absorbed cholesterol molecules themselves.

Putative prevention categories

These may be divided into two: primary prevention, where the patient is at genetic or environmental risk, but never had stones, and secondary prevention, where the patient's stones have been ablated/removed/dissolved, etc., but the gallbladder is left intact. Patients in the latter category are at considerable risk of stone recurrence since the metabolic/patho-physiological abnormalities that caused cholesterol gallstones in the first place, remain.

Primary and secondary prevention

Primary prevention will depend on identifying the lithogenic *(LITH)* genes in an individual by genotyping. Several *Lith* genes have been discovered in inbred mice, but no molecular genetic data are available in humans to date. However, as inferred from population and family studies, *LITH* genes are probably responsible for 60-80% of patients who have gallstones. Secondary prevention will depend on a knowledge of the composition of prior stones and the extent of current gallbladder function.

Murine *Lith* genes and what they do

Employing Quantitative Trait Locus (QTL) mapping, Dr. Beverly Paigen's group at The Jackson Laboratory (Bar Harbor, ME) as well as the writer's team in Boston have discovered 4 *Lith* genes in inbred mice. *Lith1* maps to mouse chromosome 2, and sister to P-glycoprotein (Spgp) is the most likely candidate protein. Spgp is now known to be the monovalent bile salt transporter on the canalicular membrane of the hepatocyte. In gallstone-susceptible mice the mRNA for Spgp is greatly increased, the expression of the transport protein is increased tenfold compared with control mice, and Spgp function is upregulated since gallstone-susceptible mice display marked hepatic hypersecretion of bile salts. *Lith2* is on chromosome 19 and the candidate protein is cMoat – the multiple organic anion transporter of the canalicular membrane. Its mRNA is also overexpressed in gallstone-susceptible mice, and its function is upregulated as inferred from the increased bile salt independent bile flow. *Lith3* is on mouse chromosome 17. Our candidate protein for this gene is Orct1, a choline transporter on the basolateral hepatocyte membrane, but its functional status in gallstone-susceptible mice is not known. We are still exploring *Lith4*, which may be located on mouse chromosome X. Our colleague, Dr. Beverly Paigen, has constructed congenic mice with *Lith1* inserted into the resistant AKR background (denoted AKR.L *Lith1^s*). This maneuver induces a phenotype essentially mimics C57L, the gallstone-susceptible mouse, especially with respect to upregulation of biliary lipid secretion and gallstone prevalence rates. Unfortunately, because we have an incomplete picture of murine *Lith* genes and their functions, and haven't yet discovered the human genes, which may be different, candidate proteins cannot at the present time be discussed as targets for gallstone prevention. Instead, we must look at our detailed physical-chemical and pathogenetic understanding of gallstone formation for more phenotypically amenable drug targets.

Cholesterol gallstone prevention: key concepts

The three concurrent biophysical abnormalities responsible for cholesterol gallstone formation prompt a number of likely targets.

– Cholesterol solubility can be targeted by stratagems that stabilize cholesterol supersaturated bile.

– Gallbladder residence time can be shortened, or nucleation can be prolonged or abolished by decreases in total lipid concentration; both mechanisms will allow solid-phase separation to occur very slowly or be inhibited.

– Altering the kinetics of nucleation and crystallization could be achieved by suppressing heterogeneous nucleation, most likely by curtailing production of mucin gel, and perhaps gallbladder immunoglobulin secretion. Decreasing the rate of cholesterol secretion into bile at the hepatic level is not proposed, since this is known to influence plasma LDL cholesterol levels deleteriously, *e.g.*, CDCA therapy.

Mechanisms and targets

Keeping gallbladder dilute, increasing bile salt hydrophilicity and increasing biliary phospholipid secretion would aim at placing the relative lipid composition of bile in a zone of the bile phase diagram known as Region E where liquid crystal but not solid cholesterol phase separation can occur. The targets for modification would be, i) inhibition of the sodium Na^+/H^+ exchanger (NHE-3) on the apical membrane of the gallbladder mucosa, ii) conversion of CDCA quantitatively to UDCA by bioengineering a subpopulation of the colonic ecosystem with an 7OH-epimerase, or by preventing secondary bile salt formation, iii) upregulation of MDR-3, the phosphatidylcholine "flippase" on the canalicular membrane and thereby increasing phospholipid secretion into bile.

Other targets could involve the gallbladder directly. They are, i) inhibiting heterogeneous nucleation and crystal growth by MUC gene suppressors, or by employing specific COX-2 inhibitors to prevent mucin synthesis, or by preventing plasma cell accumulation in the lamina propria of the gallbladder by cytokine inhibitors; ii) promoting gallbladder emptying by CCKA-receptor agonists, either by augmenting CCK release, or increasing sarcolemmal receptor response to normal post-prandial CCK levels. The latter effect could be achieved serendipitously by keeping gallbladder bile dilute.

Potential mechanisms in terms of feasibility

In Number 1, we could bioengineer colonic microbes to quantitatively convert CDCA into UDCA. There is actually an experiment of nature in this regard. Patients with Crohn's disease spontaneously acquire much higher UDCA levels in bile than the 1-2% present in health. In Number 2, secondary bile salt (deoxycholate and lithocholate) elimination from bile might be achieved with selective bacterial bile salt-uptake blockers, *i.e.*, not necessarily *via* antibiotics. Also, a new generation of bile salt sequestrants that bind hydrophobic primary and secondary bile salts selectively may be deployed successfully in this connection. In Number 3, gallbladder bile could be kept as dilute as hepatic bile, *i.e.*, ≈ 3 g/dL. This might be achieved by selective inhibition of Na^+/H^+ exchanger isoform number 3 (NHE-3), possibly by using a functional choleretic group covalently linked to one of the hydroxyl groups of the bile salt molecule. However, NHE-3 is also the major isoform of the sodium-proton exchanger on the mucosal surface of the small intestine, which may lead to untoward side effects. In Number 4, prevention of mucin hypersecretion by the gallbladder employing a potent NSAID. Acetylsalicylic acid has proven to be antinucleating in lithogenic prairie dogs and humans, but much more specific and potent COX-2 inhibitors will be reaching the market soon. It is unknown presently how one might influence MUC gene expression selectively in the gallbladder mucosa. The Number 5 approach will depend on whether *Lith1* (? Spgp) in mice is the same as the major gallstone gene *(LITH1)* in humans. If so, we could target SPGP or perhaps cholangiocytic IBAT for inhibition, and in this manner, modulate (up or down) bile salt secretion into the intestine without engendering an amplification of biliary cholesterol secretion or intestinal cholesterol absorption. In Number 6, we could enhance gallbladder emptying *via* CCK-A agonists. This will depend on safe, inexpensive CCK-A agonists and perhaps their temporary use during pregnancy to avoid third-trimester "biliary" sludge. Number 7 involves induction of biliary phosphatidylcholine hypersecretion. This might be approached by gene therapy to increase the compliment of MDR-3 "flippase" molecules on the canalicular membrane, or increasing activity of the normal "flippase" transporters themselves. In rodents, "fibrates" induce Mdr-2 gene expression, and hypersecretion of biliary phospholipid (and cholesterol), but the writer favors the porcine bile salt, taurodeoxycholate, as the most potent way to induce biliary lecithin hypersecretion, occurring perhaps by Mdr2 upregulation. It would be interesting to discover whether other hydrophilic 6α hydroxylated bile salts have the same action.

The "bile" phase diagram

Hypersecretion of biliary phosphatidylcholine, increasing the hydrophilicity of the bile salt pool and keeping bile dilute changes lithogenic bile compositions on the bile phase diagram advantageously. Normally, concentrated lithogenic bile falls into a two- or three-phase region where solid cholesterol crystallization is the end result of several phase transitions. With the aforementioned maneuvers, the relative lipid composition of bile will plot within a two-phase region known as Region E, where bile can phase-separate liquid crystals, but these can go no further toward solid crystallization.

Physical-chemical consequences of keeping bile in phase region E

Under the condition, i) the relative bile composition plots in a two-phase region where solid crystallization is a forbidden phase transition at equilibrium. ii) Hepatic bile, which normally falls in this zone, is composed of micelles plus unilamellar vesicles; but because of dilution, these vesicles fuse into multilamellar vesicles (lamellar liquid crystals) slowly and infrequently. iii) If concentrated gallbladder bile plots in this zone, unilamellar vesicles aggregate to form multilamellar vesicles (liquid crystals) rapidly, but solid cholesterol crystals will not phase separate from these.

Putative biological consequences of keeping supersaturated bile as a micellar plus liquid crystalline system

– The first consequence is that the physical state may increase gallbladder motility. It is possible that cholesterol molecules will not be absorbed or will actually desorb from the gallbladder mucosa and become resolubilized in the liquid crystals of bulk bile.

– Prevention of an inflammatory reaction in the lamina propria of the gallbladder. This sterile inflammatory response, which may also depend on cholesterol absorption from the gallbladder lumen, might be prevented by the bulk liquid crystalline state.
– Additionally, if bile is kept dilute, increased enterohepatic cycling of bile salts may result because hepatic bile will bypass a gallbladder that is full to capacity.

Can cholesterol gallstones be prevented?

Returning to the title question-clearly "Yes". It could be achieved in 10-20 years. This will be 12-15,000 years after genetic drift in our forebears in Beringia (and present-day Scandinavia and Switzerland) allowed "thrifty" *LITH* genes to dominate in our genomes. Most gallstone genes in the Western world may have emerged during the last glacial epoch, and in many ways gallstone genes, like obesity and non-insulin dependant diabetes mellitus (NIDDM) genes, are a window to this prehistoric past. Possibilities for prevention now depend on current knowledge. However, once all of the human *LITH* genes are identified, cloned, and their functions elucidated, then more rational targets will become available for pre-stone diagnosis and gallstone prevention.

Bibliography

1. Apstein MD, Carey MC. Pathogenesis of cholesterol gallstones: a parsimonious hypothesis. *Eur J Clin Invest* 1996; 26: 343-52.
2. Carey MC, LaMont JT. Cholesterol gallstone formation 1. Physical-chemistry of bile and biliary lipid secretion. *Prog Liver Dis* 1992; 10: 139-63.
3. Carey MC. Pathogenesis of cholesterol and pigment gallstones: some radical new concepts. In: Gerok W, Loginov AS, Pokrowski VI, eds. *New Trends in Hepatology 1996*. Dordrecht: Kluwer, 1997: 64-83.
4. Gerloff T, Stieger B, Hagenbuch B, Madon J, Landmann L, Roth J, Hofmann AF, Meier PJ. The sister of P-glycoprotein represents the canalicular bile salt export pump of mammalian liver. *J Biol Chem* 1998; 273: 10046-50.
5. Khanuja B, Cheah YC, Hunt M, Nishina PM, Wang DQH, Chen HW, Billheimer JT, Carey MC, Paigen B. *Lith1*, a major gene affecting cholesterol gallstone formation among inbred strains of mice. *Proc Natl Acad Sci USA* 1995; 92: 7729-33.
6. Lammert F, Wang DQH, Nelson HM, Beier DR, Cohen DE, Lecureur V, Schuetz J, Carey MC, Paigen B. Sister to P-glycoprotein is the candidate gene for *Lith1* that causes cholesterol cholelithiasis in inbred mice. 1998 (submitted).
7. LaMont JT, Carey MC. Cholesterol gallstone formation. 2. Pathobiology and pathomechanics. *Prog Liver Dis* 1992; 10: 165-91.
8. Miguel JF, Covarrubias C, Villaroel L, Mingrone G, Greco AV, Puglielli L, Carvallo P, Marshall G, del Pino G, Nervi F. Genetic epidemiology of cholesterol cholelithiasis among Chilean Hispanics, Amerindians and Maoris. *Gastroenterology* 1998 (in press).
9. Van der Linden W. Genetic factors in gallstone disease. *Clin Gastroenterol* 1973; 2: 603-14.

10. Wang DQH, Carey MC. Complete mapping of crystallization pathways during cholesterol precipitation from model bile: influence of physical-chemical variables of pathophysiological-relevance and identification of a stable liquid crystalline state in cold, dilute and hydrophilic bile salt-containing systems. *J Lipid Res* 1996; 37: 606-30.
11. Weiss KM, Ferrell RE, Hanis CL, Styne PN. Genetics and epidemiology of gallbladder disease in New World native peoples. *Am J Human Genet* 1984; 38: 1259-87.

Gastroenterology and Hepatology. The next Millenium.
G.N.J. Tytgat, G.J. Krejs, eds. John Libbey Eurotext, Paris © 1998, pp. 45-57.

Drug therapy of Crohn's disease in the year 1998

C. van Montfrans, S.J.H. van Deventer

Laboratory of Experimental Internal Medicine, Academic Medical Center, Amsterdam, the Netherlands

Crohn's disease is an inflammatory chronic disorder of the digestive tract with a predilection for the ileum and the colon. The disease may also affect any other part of the gut and cause extra-intestinal complications. The aetiology is unknown, and at present the primary goal of therapy is to eliminate symptoms and maintain the general well being of the patients, with as few side-effects as possible.
Since the publication by the National Co-operative Crohn's Disease Study Group in 1979, corticosteroids remain the cornerstone of conventional treatment of active Crohn's disease [1]. However, our knowledge of the pathophysiologic mechanisms has improved and recent data suggest that an impairment of an effective down-regulation of pro-inflammatory cytokines by mucosal T lymphocytes is central in the pathophysiology of Crohn's disease [2-4]. Therefore, new therapies focus on more specific immune suppression.
This review briefly summarizes the currently used drug therapies for active Crohn's disease and for remission maintenance *(table I)*. Some remarks will be made on the therapeutic potential of new cytokine based intervention strategies. For a more extensive discussion of medical treatment of Crohn's disease, we refer to reviews published elsewhere [5, 6].

Criteria for disease activity and remission

The clinical activity for Crohn's disease is often quantified using the Crohn's Disease Activity Index (CDAI) [7, 8]. The CDAI is a weighed score of clinical symptoms, complications and laboratory parameters. Index values of 150 and below are associated with remission; values above that indicate active disease, and values above 300 are seen with severe active disease. Most studies on the medical treatment of Crohn's disease have used the CDAI as a major endpoint. The CDAI score correlates well with quality of life indices, but not with endoscopic findings: patients with a low CDAI value may have considerable endoscopic abnormalities, and vice versa. Several therapies that effectively decrease the CDAI have only minor effects on endoscopic findings.

Table I. Guidelines for medical treatment of Crohn's disease

Condition	Therapy
I. Active terminal ileitis	
Moderately active (CDAI 150-250)	Budesonide 9 mg, 4-6 weeks
Active (CDAI > 250)	Prednisone 40 mg, 4-6 weeks, then taper in 4-6 weeks
Stenosis, big infiltrate, abscess, entero-enteral fistulae	Surgical resection
II. Active colitis	Prednisone 40 mg, 4-6 weeks, then taper in 4-6 weeks
III. Remission	
Induced by drug	No treatment or azathioprine 2.5 mg/kg or 5-ASA 3 g/day, in case of terminal ileitis
Postoperative remission	No treatment or 5-ASA 3 g/day or azathioprine 2.5 mg/kg
IV. Steroid refractory disease	
Moderately active	Add: Azathioprine 2.5 mg/kg
Active	Add: Azatrioprine 2.5 mg/kg or methotrexate 25 mg/week i.m.

Corticosteroids

Corticosteroids have a broad spectrum of action and in addition to the direct on immune cell traffic and function, steroids have substantial influence on cytokine synthesis [9].

Prednisone

Treatment of patients with active Crohn's disease with prednison in a daily dose of 40 mg usually results in a rapid suppression of symptoms, and initially 60-80% of patients responds [1]. Therapy should be continued for 2 to 4 weeks, then doses can be tapered gradually in 8-12 weeks until discontinuation. If patients subsequently fail to reach a remission they are designated to be *steroid-refractory*, and patients who initially respond to steroid treatment, but who show an increase of disease activity during tapering are *steroid-dependent*. A population-based study on the outcome of steroid therapy of active Crohn's disease reported that 30 days after discontinuation of therapy a prolonged steroid response was obtained in 44% only, 36% of the patients became steroid-dependent and 20% steroid-refractory [10].

The efficacy of prolonged steroid treatment in patients with Crohn's disease in the setting of induction and maintenance therapy has never been clearly demonstrated [1, 11, 12]. Regarding the benefit of prolonged treatment of induce remission, Brignola *et al.* observed no difference between a treatment course of 7 weeks or 15 weeks (remission rate 81% and 85%, respectively). Relapse rates were high: 6 months after stopping the treatment flare-ups were reported in 50% and 52%, respectively. Hence, no evidence exists that favours continuation of low dose prednisone use during remission to reduce the risk of relapse. Consequently, prednisone therapy should be initiated at therapeutic doses (40 mg/day) and subsequently rapidly tapered. Indeed, prednisone may cause many systemic side effects related to the dose and duration of therapy [13].

Budesonide

Recently, new corticosteroids primarily developed and widely used for asthma (*e.g.* budesonide) have been found to reduce systemic side effects. Budesonide has high topical anti-inflammatory activity and low systemic availability because of its high affinity to the steroid receptor and rapid hepatic conversion to metabolites with minimal steroid activity [14, 15].

Different formulations of oral budesonide have been developed: The first has a time-dependent and pH-dependent delivery system, *e.g.* controlled ileal release (CIR, Entocort®), to prevent absorption in the stomach and proximal small bowel. The topical uptake of this drug in the distal ileum and the caecum is approximately 70%, making it appropriate for treatment of active distal and/or right sided colonic Crohn's disease [16]. The second formulation, eudragit covered budesonide (Budenofalk®), is an oral pH modified release budenside designed to deliver the drug to the colon (approximately 40% reaches the colon) [17].

The ability of CIR budesonide to induce remission in active Crohn's disease was evaluated in several controlled clinical trials [18-20]. No statistical difference in overall remission rate was seen comparing budesonide CIR 9 mg/day to prednisone at 40 mg/day in patients with ileal or ileocaecal disease activity, after 10 and 12 weeks [18, 20]. In a placebo-controlled trial, budesonide CIR at an optimal daily dose of 9 mg was effective (remission rate 51% *vs* 20%; $p < 0.001$) in active ileocaecal Crohn's disease [19]. Budesonide caused less adrenal suppression than prednisone in the therapeutic dose, was well tolerated and steroid-associated side effects were less common [18-20]. When compared to mesalamine (Pentasa®, 3 g/day), budesonide CIR (9 mg/day) was found to be superior for induction of remission in active ileocecal Crohn's disease after 8 weeks (remission rate 69% *vs* 45%; $p < 0.01$) [21].

Treatment with the oral pH-modified release budesnide (3×3 mg/day) was less effective than 6-methylprednisolone (remission rate 56% *vs* 73%; $p = 0.024$) in patients with active Crohn's disease but caused significantly less corticosteroid related side effects (29% *vs* 70%; $p = 0.0015$) [22].

The long-term maintenance of remission has been evaluated for both formulations [20, 23, 24]. Patients treated with 6 mg budesonide CIR had a significantly longer median time to relapse compared to the 3 mg or the placebo groups in a pooled analysis of three similar designed controlled studies (263 vs 170 vs 154 days; p = 0.03) [25]. However, this effect was not sustained at 1-year follow-up (approximately 60% relapsed in all treatment groups). In a recently published study, eudragit covered budesonide at a dose of 3 mg/day was not superior when compared to placebo for reduction of relapse rate after one year of treatment (relapse rate 67% vs 65%), although the median time to relapse in the budesonide group was longer (94 vs 67 days) [26].

Taken together, in the current formulation (CIR) budesonide treatment is comparable to prednisone and can be recommenced as alternative for moderatly active ileocecal Crohn's disease only, especially in case of corticosteroid related side-effects. Although the role for budesonide in maintaining remission was not supported by the long-term studies, time to relapse was prolonged. Further trials need to determine if higher doses can improve the long term benefit for patients with Crohn's disease.

Aminosalicylates

The anti-inflammatory actions of aminosalicylates are not fully understood: yet, these drugs are important free radiral scavengers, reduce leukotriene production and can inhibit the cellular release of interleukin-1, all of which are likely to be important in reducing the acute inflammatory response in inflammatory bowel disease. In addition, inhibition of the chemotactic response to leukotriene B4, a reduction of the synthesis of platelet activating factor and inhibition of leucocyte adhesion molecule upregulation have been reported [27].

Sulphasalazine and mesalamine are widely used for treatment of active Crohn's disease and remission maintenance, but the therapeutic effectivity is controversial since publication of the results of several controlled clinical trials. Sulphasalazine was more beneficial for patients with active Crohn's disease when compared to placebo, but less effective than prednisone [1, 12]. Combining sulphasalazine with prednisone provided no addition benefit [12, 28].

High dose mesalamine (Pentasa®, 4 g/day) induced remission in 43% of patients with mild to moderately active Crohn's disease *versus* 18% in the placebo group (p = 0.0017), but was no better than placebo in a second, virtually identical study [29, 30].

In a meta-analysis of 5 control trials mesalamine significantly reduced the relapse frequency in patients with inactive Crohn's disease (pooled odds ratio: 0.53; 95% CI: 0.38-0.73 at 24 months). The pooled relapse-free rate in the treatment group was 84% *versus* 60% in the control group at 12 months [31]. A more recent and larger meta-analysis (15 controlled trials) assessed the effectiveness of mesalamine in maintaining remission of quiescent Crohn's disease: benefit was mainly observed in the postsurgical setting (risk reduction: – 13.1%; 95% CI: – 21.8% to – 4,5%; p = 0.0028). The risk reduction in the medical setting was not significant (risk reduction = – 4.7%; 95% CI: – 9.6% to 2.8%; p = 0.065), suggesting that mesalamine effectiveness increases in patients who had undergone bowel resection [32].

Side effects are frequently reported for sulphasalazine (20-40%), including nausea, anorexia and male infertility [33]. However, a meta-analysis reviewing the use of aminosalicylates for maintenance of remission in ulcerative colitis showed no apparent difference between the number of adverse events caused by sulphasalazine or mesalamine [34].

In conclusion, mesalamine at high doses has little therapeutic effect in patients with active Crohn's disease, and no convincing proof exists for a corticosteroid sparing effect or for a reduction of relapse rate. Aminosalicylates may be considered as alternative treatment in patients with active Crohn's disease who are intolerant to or refuse glucocorticoids.

Immunomodulatory therapy

The introduction of immunomodulatory therapy has provided an alternative therapeutic option for corticosteroids and aminosalicylates. The potential toxicity of these agents warrants careful consideration of their use by both physician and patient.

Azathioprine

Azathioprine is converted rapidly to 6-mercaptopurine, and active metabolites inhibit DNA synthesis by interfering with purine synthesis. The mechanism of action of these agents involves inhibition of lymphocyte function, and in particular the activity of cytotoxic T cells and natural killer cells appears to be suppressed [35].

A recent meta-analysis determined the effectiveness of azathioprine and 6-mercaptopurine in inducing remission in active Crohn's disease [36]. The odds ratio of response (OR = 2.96; 95% CI: 1.91 to 4.59) increased after 17 weeks of therapy and onwards (OR = 3.36; 95% CI: 2.12 to 6.42). Moreover, there was a trend favouring healing or decreased discharge of fistulae, which did not reach statistical significance (response rate 55% vs 29% for placebo, OR = 4.68, 95% CI: 0.60 to 36.69). Adverse events requiring withdrawal from a trial, principally allergy, leucopenia, pancreatitis, and nausea were increased on therapy (OR = 4.14, 95% CI: 1.96 to 8.62). Side effects occur in approximately 15% of patients with Crohn's disease [37]. A deficiency of the enzyme thiopurine methyltransferase involved in 6-mercaptopurine metabolism appears to account for some of the toxicities such as leucopenia and thrombocytopenia, for which regular monitoring of blood counts are required [35]. Other side effects such as rash, fever, arthralgies and pancreatitis seem hypersensitivity reactions and usually resolve when the drug is discontinued [38-40]. The carcinogenic potential of azathioprine and 6-mercptopurine in Crohn's disease seems to be low [37, 41].

Azathioprine and 6-mercaptopurine are slow acting drugs and may require three months of treatment before onset of action [42]. Intravenous loading with azathioprine is suggested to decrease the time to response and a controlled trial is ongoing [43]. The recommended doses are 2-2.5 mg/kg/day for azathioprine and 1.0-1.5 mg/kg/day for 6-mercaptopurine.

The optimal duration of therapy in clinically responding patients has not been conclusively determined. A retrospective study reported high probabilities of relapse (> 50% of patients) after stopping treatment within 5 years. However, after 5 years of remission on these drugs, the risk of relapse appeared to be similar, whether the therapy was maintained or stopped [44]. Although these results are retrospective and based on a small number of patients, our policy is to discontinue treatment with azathioprine or 6-mercaptopurine of patients in remission after 5 years.

Methotrexate

Methotrexate is a structural analogue of folic acid, that blocks folic-acid dependent pathways essential for DNA synthesis and has anti-inflammatory and immunosuppressive effects [45]. Methotrexate may facilitate corticosteroid withdrawal in patients with steroid dependent Crohn's disease. In a small placebo-controlled trial, 40% of patients achieved clinical remission and was able to discontinue prednisone after 16 weeks of treatment, as compared with 19% of patients in the placebo group ($P = 0.025$; 95% CI: 1.09 to 3.48) [46]. Methotrexate at a dosage of 25 mg intramuscularly reduces active inflammation in Crohn's disease with 2 to 6 weeks. Oral administration may suffice when methotrexate has proven effective [47].

Because of the potential for bone marrow suppression and liver fibrosis reported in autoimmune diseases, regular evaluation of blood counts and liver-enzymes is required [48]. An increased risk of hepatic toxicity was reported in psoriasis patients, but not in patients with rheumatoid arthritis, and at present data are lacking for Crohn's disease [49]. The clinical usefulness can be limited by other side effects including nausea, vomiting, diarrhea or hypersensitivity pneumonitis [45, 50].

In conclusion, the long-term efficacy, safety and adequate dose of methotrexate in Crohn's disease still have to be determined, but at present methotrexate is a useful agent for treatment of steroid refractory patients with active Crohn's disease [51].

Cyclosporine

Cyclosporine is an immunosuppressive macrolide compound, that binds to a class of cytoplasmatic proteins (named immunophilins). Cyclosporine inhibits the activity of the enzyme peptidyl propyl isomerase of cyclophillin. Immunophilins are believed to have a critical role in transducing signals from cell surface to cell nucleus. Cyclosporine has a marked inhibitory effect on T-cell proliferation and function by way of blocking the activation of transcription of cytokine genes (IL-2, IL-3, IL-4 and IFN-γ). In addition to the effect on T-cells, the effect of cyclosporine extends to other cells of the immune system, like monocytes and B-cells [45, 52].

Use of oral cyclosporine (5-7.5 mg/kg/day) for three months indeed showed a beneficial effect in an early placebo-controlled trial in active chronic Crohn's disease (59% vs 32%; p = 0.032) [53]. However, this short course of cyclosporine treatment did not result in long-term improvement in active chronic Crohn's disease [54]. In two large placebo controlled trials low dose of oral cyclosporine (4-5 mg/kg) did not reduce the incidence of flares in patients with chronically active Crohn's disease [55, 56].

Anecdotally, intravenous administration of cyclosporine was a useful agent in the initial management of refractory Crohn's disease fistulas and in pyoderma gangrenosum, however the long-term efficacy remains uncertain [57-59]. For these indications, cyclosporine need to be dosed at rather high levels with a starting dose of 2-4 mg/kg/day intravenously or 8 mg/kg/day orally. A response is expected to occur rather rapidly (within 2 weeks). Careful monitoring of blood levels is required for oral use because of slow, incomplete, and variable intestinal absorption [60].

Cyclosporine is frequently associated with various side effects, such as dose related nephrotoxicity, hypertension and hepatic dysfunction [60].

In conclusion, at present there are very limited indications for cyclosporine treatment of Crohn's disease.

Future therapy

Recent studies have demonstrated an enhanced production of several pro-inflammatory cytokines by mononuclear cells of the intestinal mucosa in inflammatory bowel disease [2, 61-63]. Experimental models have further defined the importance of specific cytokines for the induction of mucosal inflammation, by using neutralising antibodies, or by using genetically manipulated mice with a functionally inactive cytokine gene [2, 64].

Novel intervention strategies aim at either a decrease of pro-inflammatory cytokines or increase of anti-inflammatory cytokine. Of particular interest is tumour necrosis factor-alpha (TNF-α), an important pro-inflammatory mediator of mucosal immune activation in inflammatory bowel disease [65]. More than 200 patients with active therapy refractory Crohn's disease have been treated with monoclonal anti-TNF-α antibodies in various studies [66, 67]. In the first placebo-controlled clinical trial of 108 patients, a single infusion resulted in a significant decrease of disease activity (decrease of CDAI > 70, p < 0.001) and caused transient complete remissions during the 3-month study period (41% vs 12%, p = 0.008). The highest response rate was found at a dose of 5 mg/kg, which was the lowest dose studied [67]. No important short-term side effects were encountered, however the long-term effects of chronic or intermittent use need to be determined. Preliminary results of a controlled study to evaluate the efficacy and safety of anti-TNF-α antibodies for the closure of enterocutaneous fistulae in Crohn's disease showed an impressive reduction in the number of draining fistulae (publication in preparation).

Another candidate for therapeutic suppression of mucosal inflammation in Crohn's disease is the anti-inflammatory cytokine recombinant interleukin-10 (rIL-10). IL-10 suppresses IL-10 is a potent inhibitor of activated macrophages and antigen specific T-cell activation [68-70]. A phase II dose escalating study in 46 steroid-refractory patients with active Crohn's disease indicated the safety of a one-week daily intravenous infusion of 0.5-25 µg/kg rIL-10. The therapy was well tolerated and although the study was not designed to assess efficacy, 50% of the rIL-10 treated patients *versus* 23% of the placebo patients had a complete clinical remission [71]. However, preliminary data of a controlled trial investigating the efficacy of subcutaneous administration of rIL-10 in Crohn's disease patients showed less benefit (publication in preparation).

Disadvantages of cytokine-based therapies are possible induction of allergic reactions, antibody formation to the "foreign" peptides that may lessen therapeutic effects and increased susceptibility to opportunistic infections. Finally, these therapies are expected to be quite expensive.

Conclusions

Standard therapy of Crohn's disease is based on treatment with corticosteroids, which are highly effective in abating acute exacerbations, but symptomatic relapse after discontinuation is frequent. Moreover, their long-term use is limited by side effects and lack of efficacy in maintaining remissions. Budesonide CIR (9 mg/kg), a novel formulation, is a new therapy for moderately active ileocecal Crohn's disease, being almost as effective as prednisone (40 mg/kg) with less side effects. The use of aminosalicylates is disappointing both in induction and maintenance of remission. In the past few years there has been a shift from the use of unspecific anti-inflammatory agents (corticosteroids, aminosalicylates) to the use of immunomodulatory drugs (azathioprine, methotrexate). Azatrioprine and 6-mercaptopurine are safe and effective in Crohn's disease, and are usually applied in steroid-dependent or refractory patients to facilitate steroid withdrawal and maintain remission. An alternative approach in the steroid-refractory is methotrexate, which has a more rapid onset of action, in the acute phase of Crohn's disease and subsequently taper steroids. However, long-term efficacy and safety of methotrexate remains to be determined. At present, the only indication for cyclosporine is to induce a remission in steroid-refractory patients. New immunomodulatory agents have been designed for specific targets. In particular monoclonal anti-TNF-α antibodies and recombinant interleukin-10 have shown beneficial in the clinical setting of Crohn's disease. Other interesting strategies include targeting cytokine gene transcription factors or translation factors of inflammatory mediators. Currently, a placebo controlled clinical trial investigates the efficacy of anti-ICAM-1 antisense oligonucleotides, which reduces the expression of this pro-inflammatory surface protein, in steroid-refractory patients with Crohn's disease. An exciting approach for future treatment will be cytokine-based gene therapy, *e.g.* the local delivery of regulatory cytokines *in vivo*. The main challenge for management of Crohn's disease is to develop definitive therapeutic strategies that prevent, cure or effectively maintain disease remission.

References

1. Summers RW, Switz DM, Sessions JTJ, Becktel JM, Best WR, Kern FJ, Singleton JW. National cooperative Crohn's disease study: results of drug treatment. *Gastroenterology* 1979; 7(4 Pt 2): 847-69.
2. Sartor RB. Cytokines in intestinal inflammation: pathophysiological and clinical considerations. *Gastroenterology* 1994; 106 (2): 533-9.
3. Sartor RB. Current concepts of the etiology and pathogenesis of ulcerative colitis and Crohn's disease. *Gastroenterology Clin North Am* 1995; 24 (3): 475-507.
4. Mac Dermott RP. Alterations in the mucosal immune system in ulcerative colitis and Crohn's disease. *Med Clin North Am* 1994; 78 (6): 1207-31.
5. Elton E, Hanauer SB. Review article: the medical management of Crohn's disease. *Aliment Pharmacol Ther* 1996; 10 (1): 1-22.
6. Hanauer SB. Inflammatory bowel disease. *N Engl J Med* 1996; 334 (13): 841-8.
7. Best WR, Becktel JM, Singleton JW, Kern FJ. Development of a Crohn's disease activity index. National cooperative Crohn's disease study. *Gastroenterology* 1976; 70 (3): 439-44.
8. Singleton JW. Clinical activity assessment in inflammatory bowel disease. *Dig Dis Sci* 1987; 32 (12 Suppl.): 42-5.
9. Brattsand R, Linden M. Cytokine modulation by glucocorticoids: mechanisms and actions in cellular studies. *Aliment Pharmacol Ther* 1996; 10 (Suppl. 2): 81-90.
10. Munkholm P, Langholz E, Davidsen M, Binder V. Frequency of glucocorticoid resistance and dependency in Crohn's disease. *Gut* 1994; 35 (3): 360-2.
11. Brignola C, De Simone G, Iannone P, Belloli C, Evangelisti A, Campieri M, Belluzzi A, Gionchetti P, Tampieri M, Bertinelli E, et al. Influence of steroid treatment's duration in patients with active Crohn's disease. *Agents Actions* 1992; C90-2.
12. Malchow H, Ewe K, Brandes JW, Goebell H, Ehms H, Sommer H, Jesdinsky H. European cooperative Crohn's disease study (ECCDS): results of drug treatment. *Gastroenterology* 1984; 86 (2): 249-66.
13. Singleton JW, Law DH, Kelley MLJ, Mekhjian HS, Sturdevant RA. National cooperative Crohn's disease study: adverse reactions to study drugs. *Gastroenterology* 1979; 77 (4 Pt 2): 870-82.
14. Dahlberg E, Thalen A, Brattsand R, Gustafsson JA, Johansson U. Correlation between chemical structure, receptor binding, and systemic biological activity in some novel highly active 16alpha, 17alpha-acetyl-substituted glucocorticoids. *Mol Pharmacol* 1984; 25: 70-8.
15. Brattsand E. Overview of newer glucocorticosteroid preparations for inflammatory bowel disease. *Can J Gastroenterol* 1990; 4: 407-14.
16. Edsbäcker S, Wollmer P, Nillson A, Nilsson M. Pharmacokinetics and gastrointestinal transit of budesonide controlled ileal release (CIR) capsules. *Gastroenterology* 1993; 104: A695.
17. Moellmann HW, Hochhaus G, Tromm A, Moellmann A, Derendorf H, Barth J, Froelich P, Ecker KW, Lindermann A. Pharmacokinetics and evaluation of systemic side effects of budesonide after oral administration of modified release capsules in healthy volunteers and patients with Crohn's disease. *Gastroenterology* 1996; 110: A972.
18. Rutgeerts P, Lofberg R, Malchow H, Lamers C, Olaison G, Jewell D, Danielsson A, Goebell H, Thomsen OO, Lorenz-Meyer H, et al. A comparison of budesonide with prednisolone for active Crohn's disease. *N Engl J Med* 1994; 331 (13): 842-5.
19. Greenberg GR, Feagan BG, Martin F, Sutherland LR, Thomson AB, Williams CN, Nilsson LG, Persson T. Oral budesonide for active Crohn's disease. Canadian Inflammatory Bowel Disease Study Group. *N Engl J Med* 1994; 331 (13): 836-41.

20. Campieri M, Fergusson A, Doe W, Persson T, Nilsson LG, Malchov H, Prantera C, Mani V, Om C, Selby W, Pallone F, Mazzetti M, Sjodahl R, Florin T, Smith P, Bianchi P, Lofberg R, Rutgeerts P, Smallwood R, Lamers C, Tasman-Jones C, Hunter JO, Hodgson H, Danielsson A, Lee FJ, Piacitelli G, Ellis A, Weir DG. Oral budesonide is as effective as oral prednisolone in active Crohn's disease. *Gut* 1997; 41 (2): 209-14.
21. Thomsen OO, Cortot D, Jewell D, Wright JP, Winter T, Veloso FT, Vatn M, Persson T, Nylander I, group atib-ms. Budesonide CIR is more effective than mesalazine in active Crohn's disease. A 16 week, international randomized, double-blind, multicenter trial. *Gastroenterology* 1997; 112: A1104.
22. Gross V, Andus T, Caesar I, Bischoff SC, Lochs H, Tromm A, Schulz HJ, Bar U, Weber A, Gierend M, Ewe K, Scholmerich J. Oral pH-modified release budesonide *versus* 6-methylprednisolone in active Crohn's disease. German/Austrian Budesonide Study Group. *Eur J Gastroenterol Hepatol* 1996; 8 (9): 905-9.
23. Greenberg GR, Feagan BG, Martin F, Sutherland LR, Thomson AB, Williams CN, Nillsson LG, Persson T. Oral budesonide as maintenance treatment for Crohn's disease: a placebo-controlled, dose-ranging study. Canadian Inflammatory Bowel Disease Study Group. *Gastroenterology* 1996; 110 (1): 45-51.
24. Lofberg R, Rutgeerts P, Malchow H, Lamers C, Danielsson A, Olaison G, Jewell D, Ostergaard Thomsen O, Lorenz-Meyer H, Goebell H, Hodgson H, Persson T, Seidegard C. Budesonide prolongs time to relapse in ileal and ileocaecal Crohn's disease. A placebo controlled one year study. *Gut* 1996; 39 (1): 82-6.
25. Feagan B, Greenberg G, Lofberg R, Ferguson A, Persson T. Budesonide controlled ilea release prolongs remission in Crohn's disease. A pooled analysis. *Gastroenterology* 1997; 112: A970.
26. Gross V. Low dose pH modified release budesonide for maintenance of steroid induced remission in Crohn's disease. *Gut* 1998; 42: 493-6.
27. Greenfield SM, Punchard NA, Teare JP, Thompson RP. Review article: the mode of action of the aminosalicylates in inflammatory bowel disease. *Aliment Pharmacol Ther* 1993; 7 (4): 369-83.
28. Rijk MC, van Hogezand RA, van Lier HJ, van Tongeren JH. Sulphasalazine and prednisone compared with sulphasalazine for treating active Crohn's disease. A double-blind, randomized, multicenter trial. *Ann Intern Med* 1991; 114 (6): 445-50.
29. Singleton JW, Hanauer SB, Gitnick GL, Peppercorn MA, Robinson MG, Wruble LD, Krawitt EL. Mesalamine capsules for the treatment of active Crohn's disease: results of a 16-week trial. Pentasa Crohn's disease Study Group. *Gastroenterology* 1993; 104 (5): 1293-301.
30. Singleton J. Second trial of mesalamine therapy in the treatment of active Crohn's disease. *Gastroenterology* 1994; 107 (2): 632-3.
31. Messori A, Brignola C, Trallori G, Rampazzo R, Bardazzi G, Belloli C, d'Albasio G, de Simone G, Martini N. Effectiveness of 5-aminosalicylic acid for maintaining remission in patients with Crohn's disease: a meta-analysis. *Am J Gastroenterol* 1994; 89 (5): 692-8.
32. Camma C, Giunta M, Rosselli M, Cottone M. Mesalamine in the maintenance treatment of Crohn's disease – a meta-analysis adjusted for confounding variables. *Gastroenterology* 1997; 113 (5): 1465-73.
33. Taffet SL, Das KM. Sulfasalazine. Adverse effects and desensitization. *Dig Dis Sci* 1983; 28 (9): 833-42.
34. Sutherland L, Roth D, Beck P, May G, Makiyama K. Systemic review of the use of oral 5-aminosalicylic acid for maintenance of remission in ulcerative colitis. In: McDonald JWD, McLeod R, Rask-Madsen J, Sutherland L, eds. *Inflammatory bowel disease module of the*

Cochrane database of systematic reviews. Available in the Cochrane library (Database on disk and CDROM) (1), 1997.
35. Lennard L. The clinical pharmacology of 6-mercaptopurine. *Eur J Clin Pharmacol* 1992; 43: 329-39.
36. Sandborn W, Sutherland L, Pearson D, May G, Schoenfeld P, Modigliani R, Prantera C. Azathioprine or 6-mercaptopurine therapy for induction of remission in active Crohn's disease: a systematic review. I. In: McDonald JWD, McLeod R, Rask-Madsen J, Sutherland L, eds. *Inflammatory bowel disease module of the Cochrane database of systematic reviews.* Available in the Cochrane library (database and CDROM) (1), 1997.
37. Present DH, Meltzer SJ, Krumholz MP, Wolke A, Korelitz BI. 6-mercaptopurine in the management of inflammatory bowel disease: short- and long-term toxicity. *Ann Intern Med* 1989; 111 (8): 641-9.
38. Sandborn WJ. A review of immune modifier therapy for inflammatory bowel disease: azathioprine, 6-mercaptopurine, cyclosporine, and methotrexate. *Am J Gastroenterol* 1996; 91 (3): 423-33.
39. Haber CJ, Meltzer SJ, Present DH, Korelitz BI. Nature and course of pancreatitis caused by 6-mercaptopurine in the treatment of inflammatory bowel disease. *Gastroenterology* 1986; 91 (4): 982-6.
40. Cuffari C, Theoret Y, Latour S, Seidman G. 6-mercaptopurine metabolism in Crohn's disease: correlation with efficacy and toxicity. *Gut* 1996; 39 (3): 401-6.
41. Connell WR, Kamm MA, Dickson M, Balkwill AM, Ritchie JK, Lennard-Jones JE. Long-term neoplasia risk after azatrioprine treatment in inflammatory bowel disease. *Lancet* 1994; 343: 1249-52.
42. Present DH, Korelitz BI, Wisch N, Glass JL, Sachar DB, Pasternack BS. Treatment of Crohn's disease with 6-mercaptopurine. A long-term, randomized, double-blind study. *N Engl J Med* 1980; 302 (18): 981-7.
43. Sandborn WJ, Van OE, Zins BJ, Tremaine WJ, Mays DC, Lipsky JJ. An intravenous loading dose of azatrioprine decreases the time to response in patients with Crohn's disease. *Gastroenterology* 1995; 109 (6): 1808-17.
44. Bouhnik Y, Lemann M, Mary JY, Scemama G, Tai R, Matuchansky C, Modigliani R, Rambaud JC. Long-term follow-up of patients with Crohn's disease treated with azathioprine or 6-mercaptopurine. *Lancet* 1996; 347 (8996): 215-9.
45. Sandborn WJ. A review of immune modifier therapy for inflammatory bowel disease: azathioprine, 6-mercaptopurine, cyclosporine, and methotrexate. *Am J Gastroenterol* 1996; 91 (3): 423-33.
46. Feagan BG, Rochon J, Fedorak RN, Irvine EJ, Wild G, Sutherland L, Steinhart AH, Greenberg GR, Gillies R, Hopkins M, *et al.* Methotrexate for the treatment of Crohn's disease. The North American Crohn's Study Group Investigators. *N Engl J Med* 1995; 332 (5): 292-7.
47. Moshkowitz M, Oren R, Tishler M, Konikoff FM, Graff E, Brill S, Yaron M, Gilat T. The absorption of low-dose methotrexate in patients with inflammatory bowel disease. *Aliment Pharmacol Ther* 1997; 11 (3): 569-73.
48. Weinblatt ME. Methotrexate for chronic diseases in adults. *N Engl J Med* 1995; 332 (5): 330-1.
49. Hassan W. Methotrexate and liver toxicity: role of surveillance liver biopsy. Conflict between guidelines for rheumatologists and dermatologists. *Ann Rheum Dis* 1996; 55 (5): 273-5.
50. Alarcon GS, Kremer JM, Macaiuso M, Weinblatt ME, Cannon GW, Palmer WR, St Clair EW, Sundy JS, Alexander RW, Smith GJ, Axiotis CA. Risk factors for methotrexate-induced lung injury in patients with rheumatoid arthritis. A multicenter, case-control study. Methotrexate-Lung Study Group. *Ann Intern Med* 1997; 127 (5): 356-64.

51. Bologna C, Picot MC, Jorgensen C, Viu P, Verdier R, Sany J. Study of eight cases of cancer in 426 rheumatoid arthritis patients treated with methotrexate. *Ann Rheum Dis* 1997; 56 (2): 97-102.
52. Kahan BD. Cyclosporine. *N Engl J Med* 1989; 321 (25): 1725-38.
53. Brynskov J, Freund L, Rasmussen SN, Lauritsen K, de Muckadell OS, Williams N, Mac Donald AS, Tanton R, Molina F, Campanini MC, et al. A placebo-controlled, double-blind, randomized trial of cyclosporine therapy in active chronic Crohn's disease. *N Engl J Med* 1989; 321 (13): 845-50.
54. Brynskov J, Freund L, Norby Rasmussen S, Lauritsen K, Schaffalitzky de Muckadell O, Williams CN, Mac Donald AS, Tanton R, Molina F, Campanini MC, et al. Final report on a placebo-controlled, double-blind, randomized, multicentre trial of cyclosporin treatment in active chronic Crohn's disease. *Scand J Gastroenterol* 1991; 26 (7): 689-95.
55. Feagan BG, McDonald JW, Rochon J, Laupacis A, Fedorak RN, Kinnear D, Saibil F, Groll A, Archambault A, Gillies R, et al. Low-dose cyclosporine for the treatment of Crohn's disease. The Canadian Crohn's Relapse Prevention Trial Investigator. *N Engl J Med* 1994; 330 (26): 1846-51.
56. Stange EF, Modigliani R, Pena AS, Wood AJ, Feutren G, Smith PR. European trial of cyclosporine in chronic active Crohn's disease: a 12-month study. The European Study Group. *Gastroenterology* 1995; 109 (3): 774-82.
57. Present DH, Lichtiger S. Efficacy of cyclosporine in treatment of fistula of Crohn's disease. *Dig Dis Sci* 1994; 39 (2): 374-80.
58. Hanauer SB, Smith MB. Rapid closure of Crohn's disease fistulas with continuous intravenous cyclosporin A. *Am J Gastroenterol* 1993; 88 (5): 646-9.
59. Egan LJ, Sandborn WJ, Tremaine WJ. Clinical outcome following treatment of refractory inflammatory and fistulizing Crohn's disease with intravenous cyclosporine. *Am J Gastroenterol* 1998; 93 (3): 442-8.
60. Kahan BD, Welsh M, Rutzky LP. Challenges in cyclosporine therapy: the role of therapeutic monitoring by area under the curve monitoring. *Ther Drug Monitor* 1995; 17 (6): 621-4.
61. Pullman WE, Elsbury S, Kobayashi M, Hapel AJ, Doe WF. Enhanced mucosal cytokine production in inflammatory bowel disease. *Gastroenterology* 1992; 102 (2): 529-37.
62. Stevens C, Walz G, Singaram C, Lipman ML, Zanker B, Muggia A, Antonioli D, Peppercorn MA, Strom TB. Tumor necrosis factor-alpha, interleukin-1beta, and interleukin-6 expression in inflammatory bowel disease. *Dig Dis Sci* 1992; 37 (6): 818-26.
63. Brynskov J, Tvede N, Andersen CB, Vilien M. Increased concentrations of interleukin-1beta, interleukin-2, and soluble interleukin-2 receptors in endoscopical mucosal biopsy specimens with active inflammatory bowel disease. *Gut* 1992; 33 (1): 55-8.
64. Elson CO, Sartor RB, Tennyson GS, Riddell RH. Experimental models of inflammatory bowel disease. *Gastroenterology* 1995; 109 (4): 1344-67.
65. Van Deventer SJH. Tumour necrosis factor and Crohn's disease. *Gut* 1997; 40 (4): 443-8.
66. Van Dullemen HM, Van Deventer SJH, Hommes DW, Bijl HA, Jansen J, Tytgat GNJ, Woody J. Treatment of Crohn's disease with anti-tumor necrosis factor chimeric monoclonal antibody (cA2). *Gastroenterology* 1995; 109 (1): 129-35.
67. Targan SR, Hanauer SB, Van Deventer SJH, Mayer L, Present DH, Braakman T, Dewoody KL, Schaible TF, Rutgeerts PJ. A short-term study of chimeric monoclonal antibody cA2 to tumor necrosis factor alpha for Crohns-disease. *N Engl J Med* 1997; 337 (15): 1029-35.
68. Fiorentino DF, Zlotnik A, Mosmann TR, Howard M, Og A. IL-10 inhibits cytokines production by activated macrophages. *J Immunol* 1991; 147 (1): 3815-22.

69. Fiorentino DF, Zlotnik A, Vieira P, Mosmann TR, Howard M, Moore KW, Og A. IL-10 acts on the antigen-presenting cell to inhibit cytokine production by Th1 cells. *J Immunol* 1991; 146 (10): 3444-51.
70. Goldman M, Stordeur P. Interleukin-10 as an anti-stress cytokine. *Eur Cytokine Network* 1997; 8 (3): 301-2.
71. Van Deventer SJH, Elson CO, Fedorak RN. Multiple doses of intravenous interleukin-10 in steroid-refractory Crohn's disease. Crohn's Disease Study Group. *Gastroenterology* 1997; 113 (2): 383-9.

What should the clinician know about the cytochromes P450 system?

J.-P. Benhamou

Hôpital Beaujon, Clichy, France

What should the clinician know about the cytochromes P450 system? A clinician oriented to liver diseases must know few but important points concerning the cytochromes P450 system.

General considerations on the evolution of cytochromes P450

The evolutionary history of the cytochromes P450 system is a fairy tale. For a billion years, animals have been subjected to a relentless form of biological warfare waged by the plants that they ingested. As these plants progressively developed, they produced new toxins [1]. Many of these plant-derived toxins were fat-soluble and therefore could not be excreted in urine or bile. Clearly, animals which could develop systems able to transform this fat-soluble xenobiotics into water-soluble metabolite which could be excreted in urine or bile benefited from an important selective advantage. This evolutionary pressure probably explains the development of the cytochromes P450 system which metabolizes xenobiotics. By duplication of an ancestral cytochrome P450 gene, divergent evolution of these two genes and so forth (duplication follow-up by gene divergences), surviving animals have been endowed with a wide panoply of cytochromes P450 that are able to metabolize and eliminate almost all fat-soluble environmental xenobiotics, including most presently used drugs.

Cytochromes P450 and xenobiotic metabolism

Xenobiotics

Xenobiotics are foreign chemical compounds: drugs or substances contained in food or present in the environment. Most of the xenobiotics are fat-soluble and, therefore, cannot be eliminated into the bile and/or the urine without chemical changes. The animals have many enzymatic systems that are able to convert the fat-soluble xenobiotics into water-soluble metabolites which can then be eliminated into the bile or urine. Among the multiple enzymatic systems participating in this biotransformation, the role of cytochromes P450 is specially important.

Structure and function of cytochromes P450

Cytochromes P450 consist of an apoprotein with a slit, in which the substrate is fixed, and a hem. The role of cytochromes P450 is to catalyze monooxidation, *i.e.* the insertion of an oxygen atom in the substrate from molecular oxygen which is fixed by the hem. This monooxidation results in the formation of non toxic, water-soluble, metabolites. These monooxidized metabolites are frequently conjugated (sulfoconjugated or glucuronoconjugated); these conjugated, monooxidized metabolites are still more water-soluble than metabolites that are simply monooxidized. The enzymes that catalyze monooxidation are named phase I enzymes and those catalyzing conjugation are named phase II enzymes.

Most of cytochromes P450 are located in the liver, more precisely in the hepatocytes. The hepatic cytochromes P450 are in a strategic position to exert their function. The fenestrations of the endothelial sinusoidal lining allow drugs to diffuse into the space of Disse and then into the hepatocyte. In the hepatocytes, the cytochromes P450 convert the xenobiotics into water-soluble metabolites which are eliminated either into the bile, or which diffuse into the blood and are then eliminated by the kidney into the urine.

Cytochromes P450 and drug-induced hepatotoxicity

The development of the hepatic cytochromes P450 system as a means to eliminate xenobiotics has a major drawback: although most xenobiotics are transformed by cytochromes P450 into stable metabolites, other are monooxidised into unstable, chemically reactive intermediates. These unstable metabolites covalently bind to the macromolecules of the hepatocytes [2]. The effect of this covalent binding is either the inhibition of the functions of the target macromolecule or the formation of a neoantigen against which an immune reaction is mounted.

Thus, there are two mechanisms for drug-induced hepatotoxicity: metabolite-mediated liver injury and immune-induced liver injury. In the former, hepatotoxicity is increased by administration of large dose of the responsible drug; hepatotoxicity is increased by inducers of cytochromes P450; there are no extrahepatic manifestation of hypersensitivity (eosinophilia, rash, glomerulitis); if drug is readministered, the delay to the onset of liver injury is shorter than after the first administration. An example, is represented by isoniazid-induced hepatitis [3].

On the contrary, in the latter, hepatotoxicity is not independent of the dosage of the responsible drug; hepatotoxicicy is not increased by inducers of cytochromes P450; there are often extrahepatic manifestations of hypersensitivity; readministration of the drug results in a recurrence of liver injury in a delay shorter than after the first administration of the drug.

Principal families of cytochromes P450

The cytochromes P450 belong to a single superfamily of genes. The cytochromes P450 differ by the structure of their apoprotein and can be classified into 4 families (1, 2, 3, 4); each family comprises subfamilies (A, B, C, D, E, F, G), each subfamily can comprise subtypes. Over 20 different cytochromes P450 have been identified in human liver. The human cytochromes P450 that are important in drug metabolism are members of three distinct families termed cytochrome P450 1, cytochrome P450 2, cytochrome P450 3 *(table I)*.

A main characteristic of cytochromes P450 is that the activity of the enzymes is not selective, each isoform being able to monooxidize a more or less wide set of substances.

Table I. Characteristics of some human liver cytochromes P450

Cytochromes P450	Substrate	Inducers
1A2	Caffeine	Cigarette smoke
2C	Tienilic acid	
2D	Debrisoquine Most beta blockers Most neuroleptics	
2E1	Acetaminophen Ethanol	Ethanol Ethanol
3A	Ketoconazole Lidocaine Estrogens Isoniazid Cyclosporine A Erythromycin	Glucocorticoids Rifampicin Rifampicin

Intrahepatocytic location of cytochromes P450

The cytochromes P450 are particularly abundant in the liver cells. In the liver cells as compared with the cells of other tissues. In the liver cell cytochromes P450 are located in the outer membrane of the smooth endoplasmic reticulum.

Small amounts of cytochromes P450 are present in the plasma membrane of the liver cells: the cytochromes P450 inserted in the plasma membrane of the hepatocytes play an important role in the mechanism of some immunologic liver injury [4].

Small amounts of cytochromes P450 are also present in extrahepatic tissue, in particular in the kidneys.

Factors influencing the activity of cytochromes P450

Numerous factors increase or decrease the activity of cytochromes P450.

The activity of the different cytochromes P450 depends on different genes. Thus, there is a deficiency in cytochrome P450 2D6 in 6% of Western individuals and in 3% of the Asian individuals. This deficiency has an effect on the metabolism of various drugs, in particular the tricyclic anti-depressant, anti-arythmic drugs, and beta blockers.

Several cytokines, in particular the interferons, influence the activity of cytochromes P450. In patients suffering from flue, the increased interferon production results in the transient reduction of the activity of cytochromes P450. Fasting decreases the activity of cytochrome P450. Ethanol increases the activity of cytochrome P450 2E1.

Various drugs inhibit the activities of cytochromes P450 through a mechanism of competition. Thus, troleandomycine (TAO) inhibits cytochrome P450 3A4 and the metabolism of estroprogestative oral contraceptives is markedly inhibited, with an increase risk of cholestasis.

Various drugs and chemicals induce the activities of cytochromes P450. It is important to note that the cytochromes P450 are regulated independently. For example, ethanol and isoniazid selectively induce cytochrome P450 2E1, but have little effect on the activity of the other cytochromes P450. Thus, rifampicin increases the activity of cytochromes P450 involved in the metabolism of isoniazid, which results in a production of massive amount of reactive metabolite of this isoniazid, which markedly increases the risk of isoniazid hepatitis. Similarly, alcohol increases the activity of cytochrome P450 2E1, which results in the production of large amounts of reactive metabolite of acetaminophen.

Cytochromes P450 as autoantigens

An anti-liver kidney microsomal (LKM) antibodies or an anti-liver microsomal (LM) antibodies are detected in the sera from patients with different types of acute or chronic liver disease [5]. Anti-LKM antibodies are characterized by a cytoplasmic staining of the hepatocytes and the proximal renal tubules. LM antibodies are characterized by staining of hepatocytes, but not of the cells of the renal tubule. Western blotting analysis performed with liver microsomal preparations and recombinant proteins have allowed a better characterization and a better identification of the target antigen.

Anti-LKM-1 antibodies are directed against cytochrome P450 2D6 and define autoimmune hepatitis type II. They are present in approximately 10% of adults and 30% of children affected by autoimmune hepatitis. In the cases where they are present, their titer is high. In autoimune hepatitis type I, characterized by the presence of antibodies directed to nuclei and/or smooth muscle, anti-LKM1 antibodies are absent. Anti-LKM1 antibodies are also present, at a low titer, in 2% of patients with chronic hepatitis C *(table II)*.

Table II. Anti-liver kidney microsomes antibodies (anti-LKM) and liver microcomes antibodies (anti-LM)

Microsomal antibodies	Antigen	Disease
Anti-LKM1	Cytochrome P450 2D6	Autoimmune hepatitis type 2 Chronic hepatitis C
Anti-LKM2	Cytochrome P450 2C9	Tienilic acid-induced hepatitis
Anti-LKM3	Uridine-diphosphate-glucuronosyl-transferase	Chronic viral hepatitis B-D
Anti-LKM	Cytochrome P450 1A2/1A6	Autoimmune polyglandular syndrome type I
Anti-LM	Cytochrome P450 1A2	Dihydralazine-induced hepatitis

Anti-LKM-2 antibodies are directed against cytochrome P450 2C9 and are present in tienilic acid-induced hepatitis (acid tienilic is a diuretic which has been withdrawn from the market).

Anti-LKM-3 antibodies are directed against uridine- diphosphate-glucuronosyl-transferase of family 1 and have been found in 10% of patients with hepatitis B-D.

Anti-LM antibodies are directed against cytochrome P450 1A2 and are present in patients with dihydralazine-induced hepatitis. Antibodies against cytochrome P450 1A2 are present in patients with autoimmune polyglandular syndrome type 1, an autosomal recessive disease characterized by hypothyroidism, candidiasis, and adrenal failure; in 10-15% of patients affected by this syndrome, liver disease have been reported [6].

The role of these antibodies in the mechanism of liver injury is controversial, mainly because the antibodies would have no access to their coresponding antigens which is located inside the liver cell, the endoplasmic reticulum. However, the recent demonstration that small amounts of cytochromes P450 are inserted in the plasma membrane of the hepatocytes indicates that an immune attack directed against the cytochromes P450 inserted in the plasma membrane is conceivable.

References

1. Gonzales FJ, Nebert DW. Evolution of the cytochromes P450 gene superfamily: animal-plant "warefare", molecular drive and human genetic differences in drug oxidation. *Trends Genet* 1990; 6: 182-6.
2. Pessayre D. Role of reactive metabolites in drug-induced hepatitis. *J Hepatol* 1995; 23 (Suppl. 1): 16-24.
3. Pessayre D, Bentata M, Degott C, Benhamou JP. Isoniazid rifampicin induced fulminant hepatitis: a possible consequence of enhancement of hepatotoxicity by enzyme induction. *Gastroenterology* 1977; 72: 284-9.
4. Loeper J, Descatoire V, Maurice M, Beaune P, Belghiti J, Houssin D, Ballet F, Feldmann G, Guengerich FP, Pessayre D. Cytochromes P450 in human hepatocyte plasma membrane: recognition by several antibodies. *Gastroenterology* 1993; 104: 203-16.
5. Manns MP, Obermayer-Straub P. Cytochromes P450 and uridine triphosphate-glucuronosyltransferases: model autoantigens to study drug-induced, virus-induced, and autoimmune liver disease. *Hepatology* 1997; 26: 1054-66.
6. Clemente MG, Meloni A, Obermayer-Straub P, Frau F, Manns MP, de Virgilis S. Two cytochromes P450 are major hepatocellular autoantigens in autoimmune polyglandular syndrome type I. *Gastroenterology* 1998; 114: 324-8.

The esophagogastric junction

What causes transient lower esophageal sphincter relaxations?

R.H. Holloway

Department of Gastrointestinal Medicine, Royal Adelaide Hospital, Adelaide, South Australia

Transient lower esophageal sphincter relaxations (TLESRs) are LES relaxations not triggered by swallowing *(figure 1)*. They are the most common sphincteric mechanism underlying gastro-esophageal reflux in normal subjects and the most common mechanism in the majority of patients with reflux disease. TLESRs are also the mechanism by which gas is vented from the stomach during belching and are believed to be a physiological mechanism to prevent the excessive accumulation of gas in the stomach during eating. Reflux disease is thought, in part, to represent the disordered control of these events. An understanding of their mechanisms and control is central to an understanding of the pathophysiology of reflux disease and the development of therapeutic strategies for the control of reflux.

As described below, TLESRs are thought to be mediated by a vago-vagal neural reflex arc that is triggered by stimuli in the stomach and pharynx and integrated in the brainstem *(figure 2)*. This review will outline the factors that stimulate and inhibit transient LES relaxations, the neural pathways and receptors involved and the alterations in the control mechanisms in reflux disease. Transient LES relaxations have been the subject of a recent extensive review [1].

Factors that trigger or increase the rate of transient LES relaxations

Gastric distension

The most important stimulus for transient LES relaxations appears to be gastric distension. This is evident whether the stomach is distended by a balloon, gas, or a meal, and gastric distension is probably the major factor responsible for the substantial increase in the rate of TLESRs after a meal. The most sensitive region of

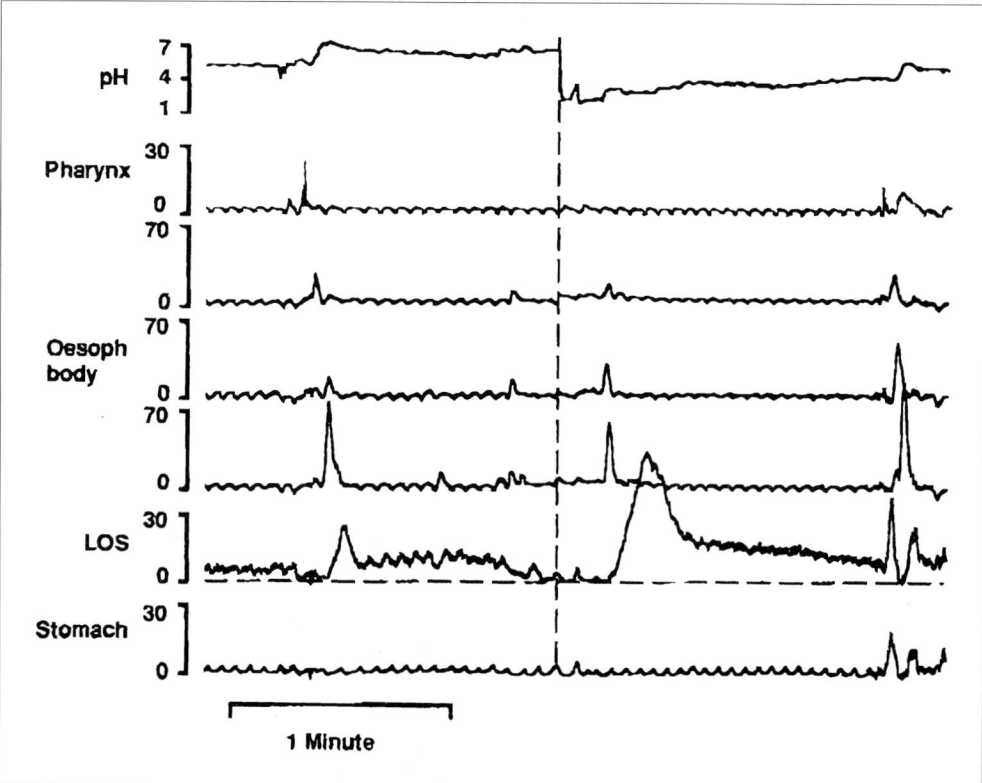

Figure 1. Example of transient lower esophageal sphincter relaxation and swallow-induced lower esophageal sphincter relaxation.

the stomach is that adjacent to the cardia. Buttressing this region with a non-expandable sleeve to prevent distension reduces the rate of gas venting and presumably TLESRs in dogs. This mechanism may contribute to the antireflux effects of fundoplication.

Food

Under normal physiological circumstances, meals are probably the major stimulus for TLESRs. The importance of specific foodstuffs, however, is unclear. Despite the clinical observation that fatty foods provoke reflux symptoms, objective assessment of the impact of high fat meals of patterns of reflux has yielded conflicting results and no significant effect has been shown on the rate of transient LES relaxations [2, 3]. Although other foods such as wine, beer, coffee, chocolate, and onions have also been reported to increase esophageal acid exposure, their impact on triggering of TLESRs has not been studied.

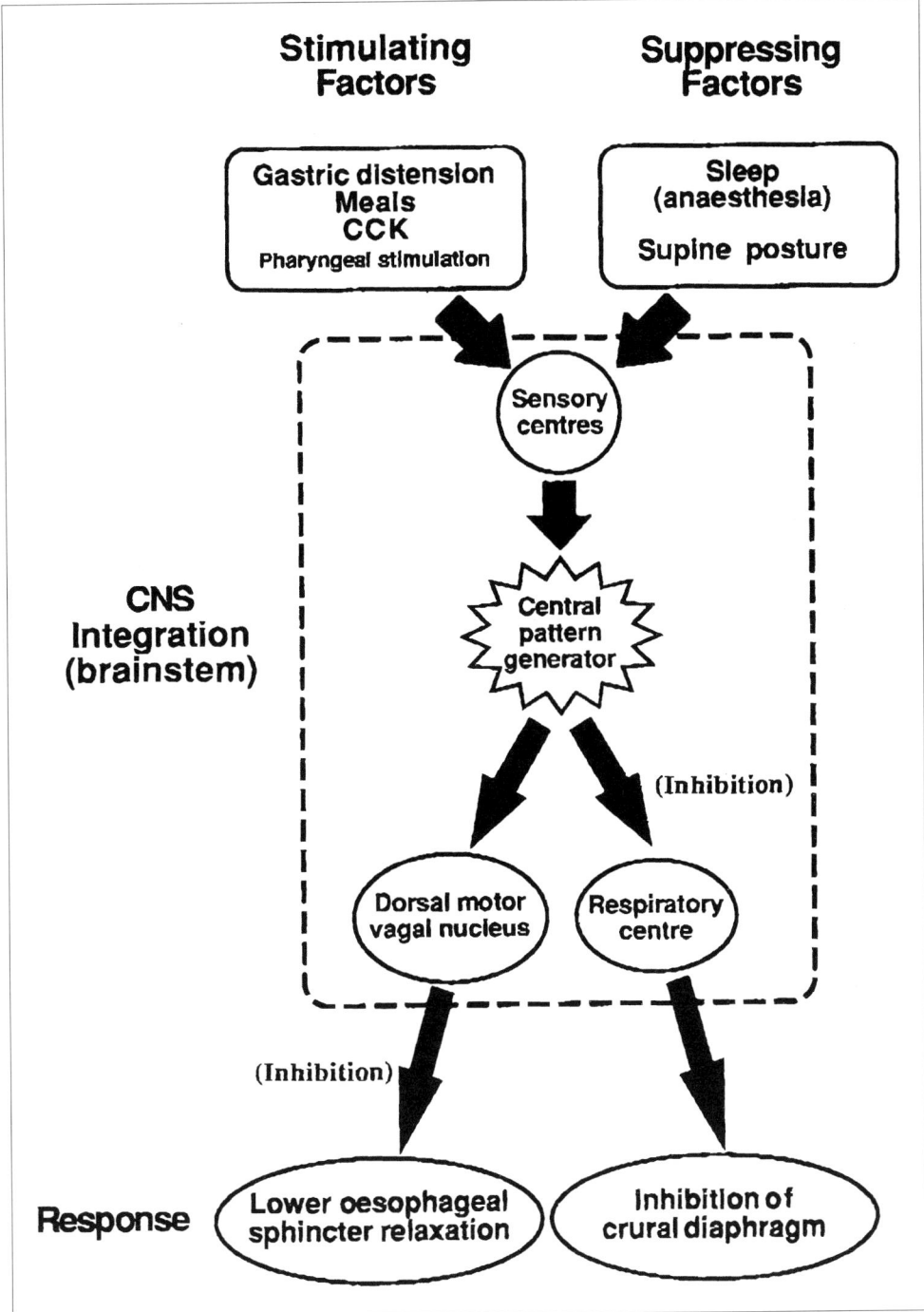

Figure 2. Schematic representation of the proposed mechanisms underlying the triggering and control of transient lower esophageal sphincter relaxations.

Pharyngeal stimulation

Pharyngeal stimulation with an intraluminal catheter also appears to increase the rate of TLESRs. Lower esophageal sphincter relaxations in the absence of swallowing can also be triggered by instillation of minute amounts of water into the hypopharynx [4]. The importance of pharyngeal stimulation in the normal physiological setting, however, remains unclear. It has been suggested that as many as 46% of TLESRs may be stimulated by subthreshold or partial swallows [5]. However, other studies, some albeit published only in abstract from do not support this notion.

Factors that decrease the rate of transient LES relaxations

Posture

Transient LES relaxations and reflux are substantially suppressed in the supine posture. The mechanisms underlying this effect are unclear. An initial hypothesis that it was due to activation of inhibitory sensory mucosal receptors at the gastric cardia by gastric liquid has not been supported by subsequent experiments in which this liquid was removed. Postural suppression also does not appear to be related to vestibular effects related to head position. Whether or not simple mechanical factors related to the position of the gastric cardia to the diaphragmatic hiatus are involved awaits exploration.

Sleep and anaesthesia

Transient LES relaxations are suppressed by sleep, and reflux and TLESRs occurring during this period actually occur during brief arousals from sleep that may be as short as only a few seconds. Transient LES relaxations are also suppressed by light general anaesthesia with barbiturates and halothane although they may still be triggered during neurolept anaesthesia with ketamine [6].

Stress

A single study has examined the effect of cold stress on triggering of TLESRs and found that this form of stress inhibited the rate of post-prandial TLESRs and gastro-esophageal reflux [7].

Neural control of transient LES relaxations

Transient LES relaxations are a neurally mediated event. They are absent in patients with achalasia. The prevailing view at present is that TLESRs are mediated largely by a vago-vagal reflex arc. Abolition of transient LES relaxations in dogs by cervical vagal cooling indicates the central role of the vagus nerve. However, the remaining evidence for the putative neural reflex pathway is largely circumstantial and has been extrapolated from our understanding of gastric and esophageal reflex vagal pathways. Gastric distension activates mechanoreceptors whose afferent nerves project to the vagal sensory nuclei in the brainstem. Activation of such mechanoreceptors has been shown to influence vagal efferent activity. Nerve tracer studies have also shown synaptic connections between motor neurons and second order neurons in the region of the vagal sensory nuclei and surrounding structures which are believed to from the basis of a central pattern generator which controls swallowing [8]. Pharyngeal sensory nerves also have their central projections in this region. It seem possible, therefore, that gastric distension and pharyngeal stimulation could trigger TLESRs by activating the central pattern generator in a manner to cause LES relaxation without swallowing. To date, however, there have been no studies that have specifically traced the neuronal connections between the gastric fundus and the nerves controlling LES function. The possibility that other neural pathways, *e.g.* spinal are involved in the triggering of TLESRs also remains largely unexplored.

The mechanism by which sleep, anaesthesia and posture inhibit TLESRs remains entirely unclear. It is possible that the conscious state influences the activity of the central pattern generator as the swallowing rate falls substantially during sleep [9].

Duration of transient LES relaxations

A prominent characteristic of TLESRs is their prolonged duration. In addition to a lack of association with swallowing, the duration of TLESRs is the other major variable that distinguishes TLESRs from swallow-induced LES relaxation. Whereas the duration of swallow-induced LES relaxation is only about 6-8 seconds, TLESRs are significantly longer and last from 15-25 seconds. The mechanism underlying the prolonged duration is not known but a long-train subthreshold vagal stimulus has been proposed [5].

Pharmacological studies

There has been considerable interest over the past 6 years in characterisation of the neural receptors involved in the triggering of TLESRs. A number of receptors have been investigated *(table I)*.

Cholecystokinin

Cholecystokinin increases the rate of TLESRs induced by gastric distension [10, 11]. The effect is mediated by CCK-A receptors as antagonism with either loxiglumide [11] or devazepide [10] inhibits the response. Cholecystokinin also appears to be involved in the increase in TLESRs associated with gastric distension and meals as these responses are also inhibited by CCK-A antagonists [11, 12]. The site at which CCK is acting remains to be determined but is probably on the afferent limb of the reflex arc as CCK binding sites are present in the afferent pathway, including vagal afferents, and in the vagal sensory nucleus and the area postrema of the brainstem. Furthermore, it seems likely that the peripheral rather than central CCK receptors are responsible for the effect as in dogs, the CCK-induced increase in TLESRs is blocked by intravenous, but not by intracerebroventricular administration of the CCK-A antagonist devazepide [10]. The response to CCK may be mediated, at least in part, by 5-HT$_3$ receptors as the selective 5-HT$_3$ antagonists ondansetron and granisetron inhibit the increase in the rate of TLESRs induced by CCK during gastric distension [13].

Table I. Receptor types investigated in the triggering of transient lower esophageal sphincter relaxations

Receptor type	Agonist	Antagonist	Effect
β-adrenergic	Adrenalin		Stimulates
Cholecystokinin-A	CCK-8	–	Stimulates
		Loxiglumide	Inhibits
		Devasepide	Inhibits
Gastrin	Gastrin-17		No effect
Muscarinic		Atropine	Inhibits
		Hyoscine butylbromide	No effect
N-methyl-D-aspartate (NMDA)		CGS 19755	Variable
Nitric oxide		L-NAME	Inhibits
		L-NMMA	Inhibits
μ-opioid	Morphine	–	Inhibits
		Naloxone	Reverses morphine
Serotonin (5HT$_3$)		Ondansetron	Inhibits
		Granisetron	Inhibits
Somatostatin	Somatostatin		Inhibits

Muscarinic receptors

Atropine inhibits the triggering of meal-induced TLESRs in both normal subjects [14] and patients with reflux disease [15]. Atropine also inhibits TLESRs triggered by pharyngeal stimulation [16]. The site at which atropine exerts this effect also remains to be determined. However, the failure of the peripherally active anticholinergic agent hyoscine butylbromide to inhibit triggering of TLESRs [17] and the inhibition of TLESRs induced by both gastric-distension and pharyngeal stimulation indirectly support a central effect of atropine.

Nitric oxide

Nitric oxide (NO) is a major inhibitory neurotransmitter responsible for LES relaxation. Nitric oxide also appears to be involved in the triggering of TLESRs. Inhibition of NO synthesis inhibits the rate of TLESRs in response to gastric distension in both dogs and humans [10, 18]. Interestingly, although NO is the major peripheral neurotransmitter in the LES, inhibition of NO synthesis decreased the rate of TLESRs but not the degree of LES relaxation thereby suggesting that, as with atropine, the inhibition was occurring centrally, possibly in the central pattern generator in the brainstem. In support of this notion, NO synthase has been demonstrated in the rat brainstem neurons controlling esophageal peristalsis [19-21].

Other receptors

Other receptors may also be involved in the mediation of TLESRs. Adrenalin increases the rate of belching in dogs suggesting involvement of β-adrenergic receptors [22]. Morphine also inhibits the rate of post-prandial TLESRs and reflux in patients with reflux disease [23]. This effect is also probably mediated centrally as, in contrast with its effect on swallow-induced LES relaxation, morphine did not affect the degree of LES relaxation during TLESRs.

Transient LES relaxations in reflux disease

Evidence suggests that there is disordered control of TLESRs in reflux disease. Although the literature is not unanimous, the majority of studies have shown that the rate of TLESRs in patients with reflux disease is higher than that in controls. Interestingly, there does not appear to be any difference in the rates between patients with and without endoscopic oesophagitis suggesting that there may be a fundamental difference in reflux disease. Also postural suppression of TLESRs appears to be preserved in most patients with reflux oesophagitis [24].

The reason for the higher rate of TLESRs in reflux disease has yet to be determined as the control of TLESRs in patients with reflux disease remains largely unexplored. One possibility is that differences in proximal gastric function are responsible. Gastric emptying is delayed in about 40-50% of patients with reflux disease. The impact of this on the rate of TLESRs has received relatively little attention but an association has been reported between the rate of TLESRs and the rate of gastric emptying in general (ref), and of the proximal stomach in particular [25]. In normal subjects, prolongation of post-prandial gastric relaxation with the 5-HT$_1$ agonist sumatriptan prolongs the post-prandial increase in the rate of TLESRs [26].

Two recent studies have investigated the motility of the proximal stomach in reflux disease [27, 28]. Patients with reflux disease do not appear to have intrinsically different mechanical characteristics of the proximal stomach that might influence the degree of stimulation to distension, and the degree of post-prandial relaxation is similar to that in normal subjects. However, post-prandial recovery of tone is delayed and is associated with increased retention of a meal in the proximal stomach. Such effects could potentially prolong the post-prandial increase in TLESRs. Other potential factors that await exploration are the impact of hiatus hernia, and the possibility that the behaviour of the gastric mechanoreceptors and/or the afferent nerves may differ in reflux disease.

References

1. Mittal RK, Holloway RH, Penagini R, Blackshaw LA, Dent J. Transient lower esophageal sphincter relaxation. *Gastroenterology* 1995; 109: 601-10.
2. Holloway R, Lyrenas E, Ireland AJD. Effect of introduodenal fat on lower esophageal sphincter function and gastro-esophageal reflux. *Gut* 1997; 40: 449-53.
3. Mangano M, Piccone A, Bianchi PA, Penagini R. High fat meals: do they really affect the competence of the oesophago-gastric junction? (Abstract.) *Neurogastroenterol Mot* 1995; 7: 273.
4. Mittal RK, Chiareli C, Liu J, Shaker R. Characteristics of lower esophageal sphincter relaxation induced by pharyngeal stimulation with minute amounts of water. *Gastroenterology* 1996; 111: 378-84.
5. Mittal RK, McCallum RW. Characteristics of transient lower esophageal sphincter relaxation in humans. *Am J Physiol* 1987; 252: G636-41.
6. Sifrim D, Miau Y, Missotten T, Ni Y, Holloway R, Janssens J. Esophageal shortening and transient lower esophageal sphincter relaxations (TLESRs) in cats. (Abstract.) *Neurogastroenterol Mot* 1998; 10: 98.
7. Penagini R, Bartesaghi B, Bianchi P. Effect of cold stress on postprandial lower esophageal sphincter competence and gastroesophageal reflux in healthy subjects. *Dig Dis Sci* 1992; 37: 1200-5.
8. Barrett RT, Bao X, Miselis RR, Altschuler SM. Brain stem localization of rodent esophageal premotor neurons revealed by transneuronal passage of pseudorabies virus. *Gastroenterology* 1994; 107: 728-37.
9. Lichter I, Muir RC. The patterns of swallowing during sleep. *Electroencephalogr Clin Neurophysiol* 1975; 38: 427-32.
10. Boulant J, Fioramonti J, Dapoigny M, Bommelaer G, Bueno L. Cholecystokinin and nitric oxide in transient lower esophageal sphincter relaxation to gastric distention in dogs. *Gastroenterology* 1994; 107: 1059-66.
11. Boulant J, Mathieu S, D'Amato M, Abergel A, Dapoigny M, Bommelaer G. Cholecystokinin in transient lower esophageal sphincter relaxation due to gastric distension in humans. *Gut* 1997; 40: 575-81.
12. Clave P, Gonzalez A, Lopez RIM, Mones J, D'Amato M, *et al.* Effect of CCK-A receptor blockade on post-prandial gastroesophageal reflux induced by endogenous CCK in healthy humans. (Abstract.) *Gastroenterology* 1998; 114: A734.
13. Rouzade ML, Fioramonti J, Bueno L. Role of 5-HT3 receptors in the control by cholecystokinin of transient relaxations of the inferior esophageal sphincter in dogs. *Gastroenterol Clin Biol* 1996; 20: 575-80.
14. Mittal RK, Holloway R, Dent J. Effect of atropine on the frequency of reflux and transient lower esophageal sphincter relaxation in normal subjects. *Gastroenterology* 1995; 109: 1547-54.

15. Lidums I, Checklin H, Mittal RK, Holloway RH. Effect of atropine on gastro-esophageal reflux and transient lower esophageal sphincter relaxations in patients with gastro-esophageal reflux disease. *Gut* 1988 (in press).
16. Mittal RK, Chiareli C, Liu J, Holloway RH, Dixon W Jr. Atropine inhibits gastric distension and pharyngeal receptor mediated lower esophageal sphincter relaxation. *Gut* 1997; 41: 285-90.
17. Lidums I, Bermingham H, Holloway R. Effect of hyoscine butylbromide on gastroesophageal reflux and lower esophageal sphincter function in healthy volunteers. *Gastroenterology* 1997; 112: A778.
18. Hirsch DP, Holloway RH, Tytgat G, Boeckxstaens G. Involvement of nitric oxide in transient lower esophageal sphincter relaxations and esophageal primary peristalsis in healthy volunteers. (Abstract.) *Gastroenterology* 1998; 114: A765.
19. Travagli RA, Gillis RA. Nitric oxide-mediated excitatory effect on neurons of dorsal motor nucleus of vagus. *Am J Physiol* 1994; 266: G154-60.
20. Broussard DL, Bao X, Li X, Altschuler SM. Co-localization of NOS and NMDA receptor in esophageal premotor neurons of the rat. *Neuroreport* 1995; 6: 2073-6.
21. Wiedner EB, Bao X, Altschuler SM. Localization of nitric oxide synthase in the brain stem neural circuit controlling esophageal peristalsis in rats. *Gastroenterology* 1995; 108: 367-75.
22. Strombeck DR, Griffin D, Harrold D. Eructation of gas through the gastroesophageal sphincter before and after limiting distension of the gastric cardia or infusion of a B-adrenergic amine in dogs. *Am J Vet Res* 1989; 50: 751-3.
23. Penagini R, Bianchi PA. Effect of morphine on gastroesophageal reflux and transient lower esophageal sphincter relaxation. *Gastroenterology* 1997; 113: 409-14.
24. Ireland AC, Dent J, Holloway RH. Preservation of postural suppression of belching in patients with reflux esophagitis. (Abstract.) *Gastroenterology* 1992; 102: A87.
25. Lundell L, Anvari M, Myers JC, Collins PH, Jamieson GG. The association between gastric emptying, gastric distension and transient lower oesophageal sphincter relaxations in patients with gastroesophageal reflux disease. *Gastroenterology* 1991; 102: A478.
26. Sifrim D, Holloway R, Missotten T, Zelter A, Tack J, Janssens J. Sumatriptan maintains the post-prandial increase in transient lower esophageal sphincter relaxations and increases gastroesophageal reflux in normal subjects. (Abstract.) *Gastroenterology* 1998; 114: A838.
27. Penagini R, Hebbard GS, Bermingham H, Horowitz M, Dent J, Holloway RH. Fasting compliance and relaxation of the proximal stomach in gastroesophageal reflux disease. *Gut* 1998; 42: 251-7.
28. Zerbib F, Bruley des Varannes S, Ropert A, Lamouliatte H, Galmiche J. Post-prandial fundic relaxation is increased in patients gastro-esophageal reflux disease. *Gastroenterology* 1998; 114: A346.

The role of *Helicobacter pylori* in gastroesophageal reflux disease

P. Malfertheiner, C. Gerards

Klinik für Gastroenterologie, Hepatologie und Infektiologie, Otto von Guericke Universität, D-39120 Magdeburg, Germany

Helicobacter pylori infection is the predisposing key factor of many gastroduodenal pathologies. Only recently it became a heavily discussed argument, if *H. pylori* may also interact with mechanisms causing gastroesophageal reflux disease (GORD). The controversy could not be more accentuated, as some data would indicate rather an indifferent, others a causal or even protective effect of *H. pylori* in GORD [1]. Data supporting either one of these hypotheses are recruited from epidemiological observations, pathophysiological considerations and clinical therapeutic reports. Along these lines the analysis will be conducted in this paper.

Epidemiology: *H. pylori* and gastroesophageal reflux disease

GORD is described as any symptomatic condition or histopathologic alteration resulting from episodes of gastroesophageal reflux, whereas reflux oesophagitis is described as the subset of GORD with histopathologic changes in the oesophageal mucosa [2]. Beside these precise definitions a goldstandard for GORD measurement is missing. GORD occurs with heartburn, but may also present with variable symptoms, and can also be asymptomatic [3]. In a prevalence-study from Olmsted County, Minnesota, GORD was defined as the presence of either heartburn and/or acid regurgitation experienced at least weekly. The prevalence of GORD in Olmsted County (2,200 residents, aged 25-74 years) was at least 19.8 per 100 residents [4]. Based on the occurrence of reflux symptoms and on the use of antacids in the population the prevalence of GORD was estimated at about 10% whereas in endoscopic studies the prevalence of oesophagitis was about 5% [3]. The

1-year-incidence of GORD is at least 1.2%/year [5]. Reflux oesophagitis may also occur in a certain percentage (0.8-8.5%) of completely asymptomatic patients [6].

The prevalence of both *H. pylori* infection and GORD increases with age, but the distribution between male and female is striking: male sex is a risk factor for GORD, but *H. pylori* prevalence is equal in men and women [1, 7]. Generally there is a decline in the incidence of *H. pylori* associated diseases like peptic ulcer and gastric cancer in the Western countries which is associated with a decline in the prevalence of *H. pylori* infection. On the contrary, GORD, reflux oesophagitis and adenocarcinoma of the distal oesophagus and cardia have increased dramatically [8]. One of the examples of this relationship is the observation that African-Americans, who have a high prevalence of *H. pylori* infection, do rarely present with adenocarcinomas in the distal oesophagus [9, 10].

The prevalence of *H. pylori in* patients with GORD is highly variable ranging from a lower prevalence to an equal *H. pylori* prevalence in patients whith GORD, *(table I)*. This discrepancy is likely to be selection biased, as age and geographical variations do interfere with *H. pylori* prevalence. Mihara *et al.* found a significant lower prevalence of *H. pylori* infection in patients with reflux oesophagitis [11]. This has been confirmed in a prospective study by Werdmuller and Loffeld [12]. In studies we conducted in our center the prevalence of *H. pylori* infection in patients with erosive oesophagitis without peptic ulcer disease and in age matched asymptomatic controls was similar [6]. These results are in line with other previously reported studies [13, 8].

Table I. Prevalence of *H. pylori* infection in patients with GORD

Study	Methods	Controls	GORD	
Mihara et al. [11]	Histology, serology	70 controls (no lesion): 67% *H. pylori* positive	70 patients with GORD: 37% *H. pylori* positive	$p < 0.01$
Werdmuller, Loffeld [12]	Histology, serology	400 controls (no lesion): 51% *H. pylori* positive	118 patients with GORD: 30% *H. pylori* positive	$p < 0.001$
Hackelsberger et al. [6]	GORD: histology, rapid urease test controls: 13C-UBT	227 asymptomatic controls: 39.2% *H. pylori* positive	130 patients with GORD: 38.5% *H. pylori* positive	$p > 0.5$
DeKoster et al. [13]	Retrospective histology	119 dyspeptic, no pyrosis controls: 45% *H. pylori* positive	70 patients with pyrosis and GORD: 47% *H. pylori* positive	$p > 0.5$
Newton et al. [48]	Histology, rapid urease test	25 controls (anaemia): 36% *H. pylori* positive	15 patients with GORD: 36% *H. pylori* positive	$p > 0.5$

The assocation between the grade of oesophagitis and *H. pylori* status is also not significant *(table II)* [8]. From the epidemiological perspective *H. pylori* does not find any support as a causing agent in the pathogenesis of reflux oesophagitis [12]. Some authors of the above mentioned studies suggest that *H. pylori* infection may protect from reflux oesophagitis than contribute to its induction [8].

Table II. Prevalence of *H. pylori* infection in GORD according to the grade of oesophagitis

Study	Method	Patients	Results
O'Connor, Cunnane [49]	Symptomscore, endoscopy	93 consecutive with symptoms and endoscopic GORD; no control	No significant relation between *H. pylori* and grade of oesophagitis
Sekiguchi [50]	Culture, serology, Serum Pepsinogen I/II level	21 patients with endoscopic reflux oesophagitis	Milder form of oesophagitis in *H. pylori* infection
Cargill [51]	Endoscopy, rapid urease test	206 pediatric patients with GORD	Most severe reflux oesophagitis in *H. pylori* positive (p=0.044)

Along these lines recent data show an increase in the incidence of adenocarcinoma at the gastric cardia and in the lower oesophagus, which parallels the increase of reflux oesophagitis [14, 15] while the incidence of non-cardia stomach cancer continues to fall, which parallels the decrease of *H. pylori* infection.

Pathophysiology

The classical concept

The mechanisms involved in gastroesophageal reflux are complex and substantially based on motility disorders in the upper gastrointestinal tract. A low basal tonus of the lower oesophageal sphincter (LOS), a higher frequency of spontaneous relaxations of the LOS, a prolonged gastric emptying time [16, 17] and impaired oesophageal peristalsis [17] ultimately lead to an abnormal acid exposure of the oesophagus and eventually to GORD *(table III)*. In a multivariate analysis impaired oesophageal acid clearance and a hypotonic LOS have been identified as the two major independent pathophysiological factors for the development of reflux oesophagitis [18]. Whether GORD predisposes to reflux oesophagitis depends on the degree of impairement of the reflux barrier, as well as on intrinsic defensive oesophageal mucosal properties, the nature of refluxate and the possibility to eliminate the reflux from the oesophagus [1, 19]. Gastric acid secretion is not different in patients with reflux oesophagitis *versus* controls [20]. Risk factors for GORD and reflux oesophagitis have been summarised in *table III* and an attempt is made to quote the potential interference of *H. pylori* with the individual functions involved in the reflux barrier [1, 19, 21].

In 1995 the concept of pathophysiology of gastroesohageal reflux disease did not even include *H. pylori* [18] while the actual discussion has begun to focus on *H. pylori* in GORD [1, 19].

Table III. Risk factors for the development of GORD/Reflux oesophagitis

Risk factors	Role of *H. pylori*
Risk factors for the development of GORD	
– **Insufficient LOS**	
– anatomic insufficiency (intraabdominal position of LOS, hiatushernia)	–
– low basal tonus of the LOS (vagal neuropathia, low concentration of motilin, high concentration of neurotensin)	?
– high frequency of spontaneous relaxation of the LOS (neuronal dysregulation)	?
– a crural diaphragma	?
– neuronal or hormonal imbalance	?
– **Motility disorder**	
– impaired antroduodenal motor coordination	(+)
– prolonged gastric emptying time	±
– **High gastroesophageal pressure gradient**	
– **Exogene factors**	
– fat	
– nicotine	
– alcohol	
– NSAID	
Additional risk factors for the development of reflux oesophagitis	
– **Disturbance in oesophageal clearance**	?
– peristaltic	–
– bicarbonat of saliva/oesophageal glands	
– **Decrease of oesophageal mucosal resistance**	
– bicarbonat	
– prostaglandine	?
– EGF	
– Capsaicin	
– **Composition of reflux**	
– gastric acid	+
– pepsin	+
– ammonia	+
– pancreatic enzymes	–
– growth factors	?

Hypothetical links between *H. pylori* and the pathogenesis of GORD

Arguments for **H. pylori** *as a causal agent in the pathogenesis of GORD*

H. pylori usually colonises also the gastric cardia in addition to the distal gastric compartments. By the release of toxins and the induced cascade of cytokines and imflammatory mediators *H. pylori* may have a direct or indirect effect on the LOS and on the oesophageal mucosa [1]. Cytokines like IL1 and TNF-alpha are reported to cause an insufficient LOS due to the relaxation of smooth muscles in the gastrointestinal tract [19]. Also prostaglandins increased by *H. pylori* may contribute to lower the LOS and increase oesophageal sensitivity to acid. If the LOS is insufficient there might be a vicious cycle with reflux, induction of mucosal inflammation and aggravation of the lower oesohageal dysfunction [1].

The role of acid hypersecretion is apparently of little importance in GORD. However it cannot be ruled out that the higher secretion of acid and gastrin induced by *H. pylori* may contribute at least to some extention to the pathogenesis of GORD [19, 22]. A lower bacterial density in the cardia compared with that in the antrum and corpus is described in patients with GORD. The frequent mucosal contact with the acidic luminal contents and mechanical irritation may create an environment that is less suitable for *H. pylori* [23].

In a retrospective study we found that among patients presenting with heartburn those with *H.pylori* infection have significant less abnormal reflux parameters in the 24-hour-pH-measurement than *H. pylori* negative patients [24]. This could either be a consequence of the ammonia production by *H. pylori* or due to a genuine selection of reflux patients with less acid reflux. We hypothesised that the *H. pylori* infection increases the sensitivity of the oesophageal mucosa by the release of toxins and other bacterial products that may render afferent nerves in the oesophageal mucosa more sensitive [19, 25].

It is known that also impaired gastric emptying does contribute to the pathogenesis of GORD. However data on *H. pylori* would not support a major role of this infection in slowing gastric emptying [26, 28].

H. pylori: *a protective element in the pathogenesis of GORD?*

Severe grades of corpus gastritis are associated with lower acid output [29]. *H. pylori* may in certain conditions such as extensive involvement of the corpus mucosa reduce intragastric acidity by inhibiting gastric acid secretion. This effect could either be the consequence of inflammation due to the production of ammonia [30] or might be a consequence of bicarbonate leakage from the inflamed mucosa and intramural back-diffusion of acid resulting in more severe disease expressions in *H. pylori* negative GORD patients than in *H. pylori* positive GORD patients. Additionally gastrin, which is elevated by *H. pylori* infection, may increase the LOS in physiological concentrations and prevent patients with reduced acid output from GORD [1].

One of the most powerful hints that *H. pylori* might be a protective factor in the pathogenesis of GORD are data which show an increase of reflux oesophagitis after *H. pylori* eradication. Labenz *et al.* could demonstrate a higher incidence of reflux oesophagitis in patients with duodenal ulcer disease and previously cured of *H. pylori* infection [31, 32]. Saccá *et al.* could confirm these findings. In 276 patients with peptic ulcer and without reflux oesophagitis 169 patients were successful eradicated. Twenty-four of these (14.2%) developed endoscopically proved reflux oesophagitis within 6 months which was mild (grade 1) in all cases. None of these 24 patients was symptomatic for GORD. In contrast only two of 107 patients who failed *H. pylori* eradication (1.9%) developed endoscopically proved and symptomatic reflux oesophagitis. Hypotheses including altered eating and drinking habits that reduce lower oesophageal sphincter pressure or the interruption of chronic treatment with antisecretory drugs for peptic disease require further studies [33]. It has to be mentioned that in contrast a randomised multicenter trial program including 309 patients with active gastric and duodenal ulcer (GU-MACH and DU-MACH) who were either treated with omeprazole triple therapy or omeprazole alone could not confirm Labenz's findings. In this study the result of treatment on *H. pylori* status was assessed by histology and 13C urea breath test. Heartburn was documented at all visits (entry, 4 weeks and 6 months post therapy) and classified as none, mild, moderate or severe. There was no evidence of an increase in the prevalence, nor of a worsening of heartburn following successful eradication of *H. pylori* [34].

The role of **H. pylori** *infection in the pathogenesis of GORD. The synopsis*

The role of *H. pylori*-infection in the pathophysiology of GORD is complex and still not fully understood. It seems as if not *H. pylori*-infection itself, but the induced type of gastritis (antrum predominant or pangastritis) is the key for the development of reflux oesophagitis. If *H. pylori* induces a predominant antrum gastritis, this will lead to higher levels of gastrin, less gastric compliance and a higher sensitation of vagal nerves due to cytokines and prostaglandins. Some cytokins and prostaglandins themselves contribute to lower LOS pressure. In the end there is hyperacidity, a higher gastroesophageal-pressure gradient, lower LOS pressure and as a consequence a higher risk for the development of GORD.

If on the other side *H. pylori* induces a uniform gastritis, this may lead to hypoacidity due to multifocal atrophic gastritis, ammonia production, bicarbonate leakage and increased mucosal H+-reabsorption. Additionally in subgroups of patients *H. pylori* may induce a normalisation of a too low genuine gastrin level which leads to a regeneration of the LOS pressure. Therefore in conditions of a uniform gastritis *H. pylori* may protect oesophageal mucosa from GORD. If after eradication the stimulus of *H. pylori* infection is missing and the uniform gastritis is healing, these patients may then develop GORD.

Therapeutical aspects

From the perspective of treatment several questions have arisen:

– Does *H. pylori* infection reduce the efficacy of PPI or not?
– Is *H. pylori* eradication necessary before long term treatment of reflux oesophagitis?
– Is the eradication of *H. pylori* a risk factor for the development of reflux oesophagitis?

Does *H. pylori* infection reduce the efficacy of PPI?

Verdu *et al.* [35] first reported in asymptomatic subjects that the increase of intragastric pH obtained with omeprazole before the cure of *H. pylori* is significantly higher than 4 or 52 weeks after successful cure ($p < 0.001$). They interpreted this finding of an increased pH induced by omeprazole in the presence of *H. pylori* infection as a consequence of ammonia production by *H. pylori* [35, 36]. These original findings have been extended by Bercik *et al.* [37] and Labenz *et al.* [38] who confirmed the same effect of reduced PPI efficacy following *H. pylori* eradication in duodenal ulcer patients.

In a recent large study on 971 patients with endoscopically proven reflux oesophagitis grades II and III according to Savary/Miller who underwent 4 weeks treatment with a standard dose of pantoprazole *H. pylori* positive patients had a significantly better cure rate when compared to *H. pylori* negative patients after 4 and 8 weeks [39]. This effect could be attributed to either a higher suppression of parietal cell function or bacterial ammonia production. In contrast Schenk *et al.* found no difference in the minimum dose of omeprazole required for relief of symptoms and cure of mucosa lesions in patients with oesophagitis [40].

The evidence so far is that PPI work more effectively in patients with *H. pylori* infection.

Is *H. pylori* eradication necessary before long term treatment of reflux oesophagitis?

As reflux oesophagitis is a chronic disease and requires long term therapy to maintain the patients in remission some concerns have been brought up of a harmful effect of long term PPI in patients with *H. pylori* infection.

In the pivotal study by Kuipers *et al.* an increase in corpus gastritis and atrophy have indeed been observed in *H. pylori* positive patients treated with long term PPI [41, 42]. In this study patients were compared from the Netherlands with reflux oesophagitis and treated with omeprazole to patients from Sweden treated with fundoplicatio. After an average time of 5 years patients treated with fundoplicatio did not develop atrophic gastritis whether they were *H. pylori* positive or not. On the contrary patients treated with omeprazole 18 of 59 *H. pylori* infected ($p < 0.001$) and only 2 of 46 who were not infected developed atrophic gastritis [43]. This was interpreted as a consequence of the different *H. pylori* distribution in the stomach with an increase of the bacterial density in the fundus and corpus and a decrease in the antrum consequently to the pH-rise induced by PPI [41]. An increase of inflammatory activity and bacterial density in the corpus and fundus mucosa during PPI treatment is a constant finding reported by all authors studying this issue [45, 46]. The induction of atrophy however is highly controversial. In fact serveral methodological shortcomings were attributed to the study of Kuipers *et al.* [43]. Their findings were not confirmed in a Scandinavian group of patients with GORD treated for 3 years with omeprazole [44]. In this latter study *H. pylori* positives did rarely and certainly not more frequently develop atrophic changes than *H. pylori* negatives.

A firm conclusion from these controversies related to changes in gastral mucosa of *H. pylori* infected patients during long term PPI is not possible as many different variables come into play. As the individual course of a patient in this condition is not predictable we personally along with the Maastricht consensus report favour the eradication of *H. pylori* in *H. pylori* positive patients before the use of long term PPI [41, 47].

Is the eradication of *H. pylori* a risk factor for the development of reflux oesophagitis?

The original observation by Labenz *et al.* [31, 32] that the cure of *H. pylori* infection in patients with ulcer disease would lead to an increase of reflux oesophagitis over a period of 3 years opened an extremely controversial discussion. Some speculated that the cure of one disease by the eradication of *H. pylori* would be obtained by buying another disease, *i.e.* reflux oesophagitis. Several other studies have confirmed the observation of an increase in reflux oesophagitis and of symptoms following *H. pylori* eradication. In the meanwhile further studies involving patients with ulcer disease and non ulcer dyspepsia were followed for 6 to 12 months could not confirm the initial observation of an increase in GORD following *H. pylori* eradication [31, 34].

To end this controversy prospective and properly designed studies need to address the relationship between *H. pylori* eradication and GORD. The currently available and contrasting reports have set the stage for these studies and we need to await their results before drawing final conclusions.

Conclusion

H. pylori is a new factor to be considered in patients with GORD. There is a collection of new data which do either support or dismiss the role of *H. pylori* in the pathogenesis of GORD. The impact for clinical practice is controversial. Some recommend a test-and-treat strategy in all patients with GORD. Some advocate to preserve *H. pylori* because of its protective effect against GORD. Personally we stick to the Maastricht recommendation and consider treatment advisable for those needing long term PPI. It will be the task of future studies to provide the definitive clue of the *H. pylori*/GORD relationship.

References

1. Labenz J, Malfertheiner P. *Helicobacter pylori* in gastro-oesophageal reflux disease: causal agent, independent or protective factor? *Gut* 1997; 41: 277-80.
2. Kahrilas PJ. Gastroesophageal reflux disease. *JAMA* 1996; 276: 983-8.
3. Petersen H. The prevalence of gastroesophageal reflux disease. *Scand J Gastroenterol* 1995; 30 (Suppl.) 211: 5-6.

4. Locke GR, Talley NJ, Fett SL, Zinsmeister AR, Melton LJ. Prevalence and clinical spectrum of gastroesophageal reflux: A population based study in Olmsted County, Minnesota. *Gastroenterology* 1997; 112: 1448-56.
5. Lööf L, Götell P, Elfberg B. The incidence of reflux oesophagitis. A study of endoscopy report from a defined catchment area in Sweden. *Scan J Gastroenterol* 1993; 28: 113-8.
6. Hackelsberger A, Schultze V, Günther T, Arnim U, Manes G, Malfertheiner P. The prevalence of *Helicobacter pylori* gastritis in patients with reflux oesophagitis: a case-control study. *Eur J Gastroenterol Hepatol* (in press).
7. Buckley MJM, O'Shea J, Grace A, English L, Keane C, Houihan D, O'Morain CA. A community based study of the epidemiology of *Helicobacter pylori* infection and associated asymptomatic gastroduodenal pathology. *Eur J Gastroenterol Hepatol* 1998; 10: 375-9.
8. Xia HH-X, Talley N. *Helicobacter pylori* infection, reflux esophagitis, and atrophic gastritis: an unexplored triangle. *Am J Gastroenterol* 1998; 93: 394-400.
9. Hesketh PJ, Clapp RW, Doos WG, Spechler SJ. The increasing frequency of adenocarcinoma of the esophagus. *Cancer* 1989; 64: 526-30.
10. Graham DY, Malaty HM, Evans DG, Evans DJ, Klein PD, Adam E. Epidemiology of *Helicobacter pylori* in a asymptomatic population in the United States. Effect of age, race and socioeconomic status. *Gastroenterology* 1991; 100: 1495-501.
11. Mihara M, Haruma K, Kamada T, Kiyohira K, Goto T, Sumii M, Tanaka S, Yoshihara M, Sumii K, Kajiyama G. Low prevalence of *Helicobacter pylori* infection in patients with reflux esophagitis. *Gut* 1996; 39 (Suppl.): A94.
12. Werdmuller BF, Loffeld RJ. *Helicobacter pylori* infection has no role in the pathogenesis of reflux esophagitis. *Dig Dis Sci* 1997; 42: 103-5.
13. DeKoster E, Ferhat M, Deprez C, Delterne M. *Helicobacter pylori*, gastric histology and gastroesophageal reflux disease. *Gut* 1995; 37 (Suppl.): A144.
14. Correa P, Chen VW. Gastric cancer. *Cancer Surv* 1994; 19-20: 55-76.
15. Lord RV, Law MG, Ward RL, Giles GG, Thomas RJ, Thursfield V. Rising incidence of oesophageal adenocarcinoma in men in Australia. *J Gastroenterol Hepatol* 1998; 13: 356-62.
16. Mc Callum RW, Berkowitz DM, Lerner E. Gastric emptying in patients with gastroesophageal reflux. *Gastroenterology* 1981; 80: 285-91.
17. Lundell L, Myers JC, Maieson GG. Is motility impaired in the entire upper gastrointestinal tract in patients with gastroesophageal reflux disease? *Scand J Gastroenterol* 1996; 31: 131-5.
18. Cadiot G, Bruhat A, Rigaud D, Coste T, Vuagnat A, Benyedder Y, Vallot T, Le Guludec D, Mignon M. Multivariate analysis of pathophysiological factors in reflux oesophagitis. *Gut* 1997; 40: 167-74.
19. Mane G, Dominguez-Munoz JE, Leodolter A, Malfertheiner P. Pathogenese der gastroösophagealen Refluxkrankheit: Rolle des *Helicobacter pylori*. *Chirurgische Gastroenterologie* 1997; 13: 92-6.
20. Hirshowitz BI. A critical analysis with appropriate controls, of gastric acid and pepsin secretion in clinical esophagitis. *Gastroenterology* 1991; 101: 1149-58.
21. Wetscher GJ, Glaser K, Wieschemeyer Th, Gadenstätter M, Profanter Ch. Pathophysiologie der gastroösophagealen Refluxkrankheit. *Chirugische Gastroenterologie* 1997; 13: 86-91.
22. El-Omar E, Penman T, Dorrian CA, Ardill JE, McColl KE. Eradicating *Helicobacter pylori* infection lowers gastrin mediated acid secretion by two thirds in patients with duodenal ulcer. *Gut* 1993; 34: 1060-5.
23. Hackelsberger A, Günther T, Schultze V, Labenz J, Roessner A, Malfertheiner P. Prevalence and pattern of *Helicobacter pylori* gastritis in the gastric cardia. *Am J Gastroenterol* 1997; 92: 2220-4.

24. Leodolter A, Dominguez-Munoz JE, Gerards C, Hackelsberger A, Malfertheiner P. Impact of *Helicobacter pylori* infection on gastroesophageal reflux. *Gastroenterology* 1998; 114: A200.
25. Meyer EA, Gebhart GF. Basic and clinical aspects of visceral hyeralgesia. *Gastroenterology* 1994; 107: 271-93.
26. Scott AM, Kellow JE, Shuter B, Cowan H, Corbett AM, Riley JW, Lunzer MR, Eckstein RP, Hoschl R, Lam SK. Intragastric distribution and gastric emptying of solids and liquids in functionnal dyspepsia. Lack of influence of symptom subgroups and *H. pylori* associated gastritis. *Dig Dis Sci* 1993; 38: 2247-54.
27. Pieramico O, Ditschuneit H, Malfertheiner P. Gastrointestinal motility in patients with non-ulcer dyspepsia: a role for *H. pylori* infection? *Am J Gastroenterol* 1993; 88: 364-8.
28. Qvist N, Rasmussen L, Axelsson CK. *H. pylori* associated gastritis and dyspepsia. The influence on migrating motor complexes. *Scand J Gastroenterol* 1994; 29: 133-7.
29. Feldman M, Cryer B, McArthur KE, Huet BA, Lee E. Effects of aging and gastritis on gastric acid and pepsin secretion in humans: a prospective study. *Gastroenterology* 1996; 110: 1043-52.
30. Goggin PM, Marrero JM, Ahmed H, Jackson PA, Corbishley CM, Northfield TC. Urea hydrolysis in *Helicobacter pylori* infection. *Eur J Gastroenterol Hepatol* 1991; 3: 927-33.
31. Labenz J, Tillenburg B, Peitz U, Börsch G. Long term consequences of *Helicobacter pylori* eradication: clinical aspects. *Scand J Gastroenterol* 1996, 31 (Suppl. 215): 111-5.
32. Labenz J, Blum AL, Bayerdörffer E, Meining A, Stolte M, Börsch G. Curing *Helicobacter pylori* infection in patients with duodenal ulcer may provoke reflux esophagitis. *Gastroenterology* 1997; 112: 1442-7.
33. Saccá N, De Medici A, Rodinó S, De Siena M, Giglio A. Reflux esophagitis: A complication of *Helicobacter pylori* eradication therapy? *Endoscopy* 1997; 29: 224.
34. Malfertheiner P, Veldhuyzen van Zanten S, Dent J, Bayerdörffer E, Lind T, O'Morain C, Spiller RC, Unge P, Zeijlon L. Does cure of *Helicobacter pylori* infection induce heartburn? *Gastroenterology* 1998; 114: A212.
35. Verdu EF, Armstrong D, Idström JP, Labenz J, Stolte M, Börsch G, Blum AL. Intragastric pH during treatment with omeprazole: role of *Helicobacter pylori* and *H. pylory*-associated gastritis. *Scand J Gastroenterol* 1996; 31: 1151-6.
36. Verdu EF, Armstrong D, Idström JP, Labenz J, Stolte M, Dorta G, Börsch G, Blum AL. Effect of curing *Helicobacter pylori* infection on intragastric pH during treatment with omeprazole. *Gut* 1995; 37: 743-8.
37. Bercik P, Verdu EF, Armstrong D, Cederberg C, Idström JP, Stolte M, Blum AL. *H. pylori* related increase in omeprazole (OME) effect is associated with ammonia production. *Gastroenterology* 110 (Suppl.) A64.
38. Labenz J, Tillenburg B, Peitz U, Börsch G, Idström JP, Verdu E, Stolte M, Blum AL. Efficacy of omeprazole one year after cure of *Helicobacter pylori* infection in duodenal ulcer patients. *Am J Gastroenterol* 1997; 92: 576-81.
39. Holtmann G, Cain C, Malfertheiner P. *Helicobacter pylori* accelerates healing of reflux oesophagitis during treatment with the proton pump inhibitor pantoprazole (in press).
40. Schenk BE, Kuipers EJ, Klinkenberg-Knol EC, Eskes SA, Meuwissen SGM. *H. pylori*, GERD and the efficacy of omeprazole therapy. *Gastroenterology* 112 (Suppl.): A282.
41. Kuipers EJ, Uyterlinde AM, Pena AS, Hazenberg HJA, Bloemena E, Lindeman J, Klinkenberg-Knol EC, Meuwissen SGM. Increase of *Helicobacter pylori* associated corpus gastritis during acid suppressive therapy: implication for long term safety. *Am J Gastroenterol* 1995; 90: 1401-6.

42. Logan RPH, Walker MM, Misiewicz JJ, Gummett PA, Karim QN, Baron JH. Changes in the intragastric distribution of *Helicobacter pylori* during treatment with omeprazole. *Gut* 1995; 36: 12-6.
43. Kuipers EJ, Lundell L, Klinkenberg EC, Havu N, Festen HPM, Liedman B, Lamers C, Jansen J, Dalenbäck J, Snel P, Nells GD, Meuwissen St. Atrophic gastritis and *Helicobacter pylori* infection in patients with reflux esophagitis treated with omeprazole or fundoplication. *N Engl J Med* 1996; 334: 1018-22.
44. Lundell L, Havu N, Andersson A. Gastritis development and acid suppression therapy revisited. Results of a randomised clinical study with long term follow-up. *Gastroenterology* 1997; 112: A28.
45. Stolte M, Bethke B. Elimination of *H. pylori* under treatment with omeprazole. *Z Gastroenterol* 1991; 28: 271.
46. Logan RPH, Walker MM, Misiewiez JJ. Changes in the intragastric distribution of *H. pylori* during treatment with omeprazole. *Gut* 1995; 36: 12.
47. The European *Helicobacter pylori* Study Group. Current European concepts in the management of *Helicobacter pylori* infection. The Maastricht Consensus Report. *Gut* 1997; 41: 8-13.
48. Newton M, Bryan R, Burnham WR, Kamm MA. Evaluation of *Helicobacter pylori* in reflux oesophagitis and Barrett's oesophagus. *Gut* 1997; 40: 9-13.
49. O'Connor HJ, Cunnane K. *Helicobacter pylori* and gastroesophageal reflux disease – a prospective study. *Ir J Med Sci* 1994; 163: 369-73.
50. Sekiguchi T, Shirota T, Horikoshi T, Kawamura O, Toki M, Kusano M, Kon Y, Ohwada T. *Helicobacter pylori* infection and severity of reflux esophagitis *Gastroenterology* 1996; 110: A755.
51. Cargill G, Atlan P, Tudor D, Regnault C. Association of *Helicobacter pylori* and reflux esophagitis in symptomatic children. *Gastroenterology* 1994, 106: A59.

Inflammation and intestinal metaplasia of cardia and gastroesophageal junction

E. Solcia

Department of Pathology, University of Pavia and IRCCS Policlinico San Matteo, Pavia, Italy

Carditis

Cardia mucosa gastritis (carditis) has been reported frequently both in patients with gastroesophageal reflux disease and in patients with chronic inflammation of other gastric sites [1-3]. This arises the question as to whether carditis is merely to be interpreted as a cardia extension of *Helicobacter pylori* gastritis or may represent an independent pathologic entity related to reflux disease. To investigate this issue we performed a systematic histologic study of antral, corpus, cardia (0.5 cm below the Z line) and esophageal (2 cm above the Z line) mucosa in a series of 221 patients (mean age 53.7 ± 14.1) with reflux symptoms (with or without esophageal erosions at endoscopy), a variety of dyspeptic symptoms or no symptoms [4, 5]. The results showed correlation of cardia mucosa inflammation with *H. pylori* infection and with inflammation of other gastric sites, but not with endoscopic or histologic signs of esophagitis. In addition, a correlation of cardia inflammation with fixed epigastric (retroxiphoid) pyrosis and, less obviously, with heartburn (retrosternal burning irradiating upwards) and acid reflux (but not with dysphagia or non-cardiac chest pain) has been observed. In only 4 out of the 217 cases investigated cardia gastritis was found in the absence of gastritis of other sites. *H. pylori* colonization was observed in 123 of the 164 (75%) cases with carditis, either in the cardia itself (92 cases) or elsewhere. Most inflammatory changes of cardia mucosa in *H. pylori* negative cases resembled those of *H. pylori* positive subjects. No patterns diagnostic for "chemical" gastritis were detected.

Investigation of another series of 49 subjects (mean age 52.5 + 12.9 years, 40 with endoscopy negative reflux disease confirmed by 24 hours pHmetry and 9 controls without reflux disease) showed lack of correlation between cardia mucosa inflammation and esophageal pHmetry or histologic signs of esophagitis. It is concluded that, at least in a population with rather high *H. pylori* prevalence (153/270 = 56.7%)

such as the endoscopic patients we investigated, cardia gastritis is mostly to be interpreted as a cardia extension of ordinary *H. pylori* gastritis which for the severity of glandular involvement resembles more antral than corpus-fundus gastritis [3, 4], and, apparently, shows no relationship with gastroesophageal reflux disease. Some relationship between cardia mucosa inflammation and reflux disease has been suggested by some studies [2, 6, 7] and denied by others, who found a correlation with *H. pylori* infection [8, 9]. In addition, a correlation of short segment Barrett's esophagus with both histological esophagitis and inflammation at the gastroesophageal junction has been reported [10]. However, further systematic investigation of junctional squamo-columnar mucosa separated from short Barrett's epithelium as well as of distant cardia (0.5 to 1.5 cm below the Z line) and esophageal (2 cm above the Z line) mucosa in subjects carefully characterized for reflux disease is needed.

Intestinal metaplasia

With the alcian blue-periodic acid Schiff (AB-PAS) method intestinal metaplasia of cardia mucosa has been found in 51 of the 217 (23.5%) cases investigated, compared with 28.5% of antrum and 3.2% of corpus mucosa from the same series. Only 4 of 140 patients with esophageal biopsies showed intestinal-type Barrett's esophagus, two with and two without coexisting cardia intestinal metaplasia. The high iron diamine (HID) test showed sulphomucins in all Barrett lesions as well as in 39% of cardia and 14% of antral intestinal metaplasia. In the second series of patient investigated, intestinal metaplasia was detected in 32.7% of cardia and 36.7% of antra investigated and sulphomucins in 7 of 16 (43.7%) and 1 of 18 (5.6%) cases, respectively. Together, the two series showed intestinal metaplasia in 67 of 266 (25.2%) cardia investigated and 81 of 270 (30.3%) antra. Sulphomucins-positive type III lesions were found in 40.3% of cardia and 12.3% of antral intestinal metaplasia cases. There was a weak correlation between cardia and antral intestinal metaplasia and between cardia intestinal metaplasia and *H. pylori* colonization or inflammatory changes of cardia mucosa. High sampling error due to focality of metaplastic changes and (spontaneous or drug induced) bacterial eradication intervening after the development of these changes might account for such relatively weak correlations. No correlation was found between cardia intestinal metaplasia and either endoscopic and histologic signs of reflux esophagitis or symptoms and pHmetry suggestive of reflux disease.

Recently, a high prevalence of intestinal metaplasia of cardia mucosa has been also found in other studies using the alcian blue-periodic acid Schiff stain, instead of usual hematoxylin-eosin [11]. In addition, no correlation with Barrett's esophagus, esophagitis or reflux disease and positive correlation with *H. pylori* infection and chronic inflammation of the cardia have been found [9, 11, 12].

It has been ascertained that adenocarcinomas arising in the distal esophagus/proximal stomach differ from those arising in the distal stomach for their stronger correlation with white race, male sex, peptic ulcer, reflux disease, long and short segment Barrett's esophagus or hiatal hernia, lack of correlation with *H. pylori* infection and lack of diffuse signet-ring cancers [13-15]. However, among such adenocarcinomas, tumors arising in the cardia showed weaker correlation with race, reflux disease, Barrett's epithelium or hiatal hernia than did those arising in the esophagus [14], thus suggesting the possibility that other factors, more akin to those involved in the pathogenesis of distal gastric cancer, might operate in at least a subset of cardia cancers. Whether chronic gastritis and/or intestinal metaplasia of the cardia mucosa are involved in this process it remains to be established. A contribution of gastroesophageal reflux to chronic inflammation and intestinal metaplasia of the gastroesophageal junction and cardia has been also proposed [2, 6, 7] but denied by others [9, 11, 12]. Whatever its origin the high (around 40%) proportion of sulphomucin positive type III intestinal metaplasia found in the cardia may be clinically relevant as this type of metaplasia has been linked with cancer development [16].

The relevance and complexity of this matter is outlined by the increasing incidence of the adenocarcinoma of the cardia and cardioesophageal junction, concomitant with the decreasing incidence of distal gastric cancer, the difficulty to quantify the contribution of cancers arising in short segment Barrett's epithelium [17] and the difficulty to identify the gastro-esophageal junction at endoscopy clearly enough to separate short segment Barrett from intestinal metaplasia of the gastroesophageal junction (so-called ultrashort Barrett) and from intestinal metaplasia of cardia mucosa showing no direct contact with the squamo-columnar junction.

References

1. Fink SM, Barwick KW, De Luca V, Sanders FJ, Kandathil M, McCallum RW. The association of histologic gastritis with gastroesophageal reflux and delayed gastric emptying. *J Clin Gastroenterol* 1984; 6: 301-9.
2. Clark GWB, Ireland AP, Chandrasoma P, DeMeester TR, Peters JH, Bremner CG. Inflammation and metaplasia in the transitional epithelium of the gastroesophageal reflux disease (abstract). *Gastroenterology* 1994; 106: 63.
3. Genta RM, Huberman RM, Grahan DY. The gastric cardia in *Helicobacter pylori* infection. *Hum Pathol* 1994; 25: 915-9.
4. Solcia E, Villani L, Trespi E, *et al.* Cardia mucosa gastritis (carditis): pathogenesis, correlation with gastritis of other sites and clinicopathological relevance. In: Hunt RH, Tytgat GNJ, eds. Helicobacter pylori: *basic mechanisms to clinical cure 1998*. Dordrecht: Kluwer Academic Publishers, 1998.
5. Villani L, Trespi E, Fiocca R, *et al*. Analysis of gastroduodenitis and oesophagitis in relation to dyspeptic/reflux symptoms. *Digestion* 1998; 59: 91-101.
6. Riddell RH. The biopsy diagnosis of gastroesophageal reflux disease, "carditis", and Barrett's esophagus, and sequelae of therapy. *Am J Surg Pathol* 1996; 20: S31-50.
7. Oberg S, Peters JH, De Meester TR, *et al*. Inflammation metaplasia of cardiac mucosa is a manifestation of gastroesophageal reflux disease. *Ann Surg* 1997; 226: 522-32.
8. Spechler SJ, Wang HH, Chen YY, Zeroogian JM, Antonioli DA, Goyal RK. Inflammation of the gastric cardia and *H. pylori* infection are not risk factors for intestinal metaplasia at the esophagogastric junction (abstract). *Gastroenterology* 1997; 112: A297.

9. Goldblum JR, Vicari JJ, Falk GW, *et al.* Inflammation and intestinal metaplasia of the gastric cardia: the role of gastroesophageal reflux and *H. pylori* infection. *Gastroenterology* 1998; 114: 633-9.
10. Nandurkar S, Talley NJ, Martin CJ, Adams S. Short segment Barrett's oesophagus: prevalence, diagnosis and associations. *Gut* 1997; 40: 710-5.
11. Morales GT, Sampliner RE, Bhattacharyya A. Intestinal metaplasia of the gastric cardia. *Am J Gastroenterol* 1997; 92: 414-8.
12. Hirota WK, Loughney TM, Lazas DJ, Maydonovitch CL, Wong RKH. Is *Helicobacter pylori* associated with specialized intestinal metaplasia of the esophagus or stomach? A prospective study of 889 patients (abstract). *Gastroenterology* 1997; 112: A149.
13. Kalish RJ, Clancy PE, Orringer MB, Appelman HD. Clinical, epidemiologic, and morphologic comparison between adenocarcinomas arising in Barrett's esophageal mucosa and in the gastric cardia. *Gastroenterology* 1984; 86: 461-7.
14. Mac Donald WC, Mac Donald JB. Adenocarcinoma of the esophagus and/or gastric cardia. *Cancer* 1987; 60: 1094-8.
15. Parsonnet J, Friedman GF, Vandersteen D, *et al. Helicobacter pylori* infectious and the risk of gastric carcinoma. *N Engl J Med* 1991: 325: 1127-31.
16. Filipe MI, Munoz N, Matko L, *et al.* Intestinal metaplasia type and the risk of gastric cancer: a cohort study in Slovenia. *Int J Cancer* 1994; 57: 324-9.
17. Schenell TG, Sontag SJ, Chejfec G. Adenocarcinoma arising in tongues or short segments of Barrett's esophagus. *Dig Dis Sci* 1992; 37: 137-43.

Proton pump inhibitors or laparoscopic antireflux surgery?

L. Lundell

Department of Surgery, Sahlgrenska University Hospital, S-413 45 Göteborg, Sweden

Recent advantages in the medical treatment of gastroesophageal reflux disease (GORD) now allow the physician to both heal acute episodes of esophagitis and maintain these patients in clinical remission [1]. It is also generally accepted that medical therapy can be used as a long term maintenance therapy and may also be a legitimate alternative to surgery for the management of severe, long-standing GORD [2]. A comprehensive assessment of the relative merit of the different treatment options requires, however, a generally accepted criteria for the assessments of the severity of GORD with respect both to symptoms and/or the presence of complications. There are methodological difficulties in allowing a proper comparison between medical and surgical therapy for GORD, but the present review is aimed at assessing the merits of medical and surgical therapy per se and to put these therapeutic alternatives also into in the context of natural history and complications of the disease.

Efficacy of medical treatment

The main priority of any treatment based on a proper diagnosis of GORD is to control symptoms arising directly from oesophageal mucosal contact with refluxed contents of predominantly gastric nature. The three general classes of medication used in similar therapy of reflux oesophagitis [3] and also in endoscopy negative reflux disease are antisecretory drugs, prokinetics agents and mucosal coating compounds. There seems to be a close correlation between the degree of inhibition of gastric acid secretion and the subsequent capacity of these drugs to heal the oesophagitis [4, 5]. Consequently, the clinical experience with the most effective acid inhibitory drugs, proton pump inhibitors, reveals that there are essentially very few patients resistant to this type of medical treatment.

The success of short term medical therapy in patients with reflux oesophagitis essentially depends on two factors: one is the pre-treatment severity of the erosive and/or ulcerative lesions in the oesophagus and the other is the choice of drug therapy [6-10]. However, irrespective of the type of initial drug therapy, patients will relapse frequently after cessation of treatment. The slope of this relapse curve might be dependent on the pre-treatment severity of the oesophagitis, as well, but other factors of clinical importance may also be operating [7, 11]. The slope of the relapse curve seems to be steep suggesting that reflux esophagitis, in many cases, is a chronic disease. The number of studies reporting an overwhelming efficacy of omeprazole and other proton pump inhibitors such as lanzoprazole and pantoprazole as a maintenance therapy for reflux esophagitis is increasing [12-18]. Even in patients with more severe grades of esophagitis have these drugs been proven to be adequate in all but a minority of patients *(figure 1)*.

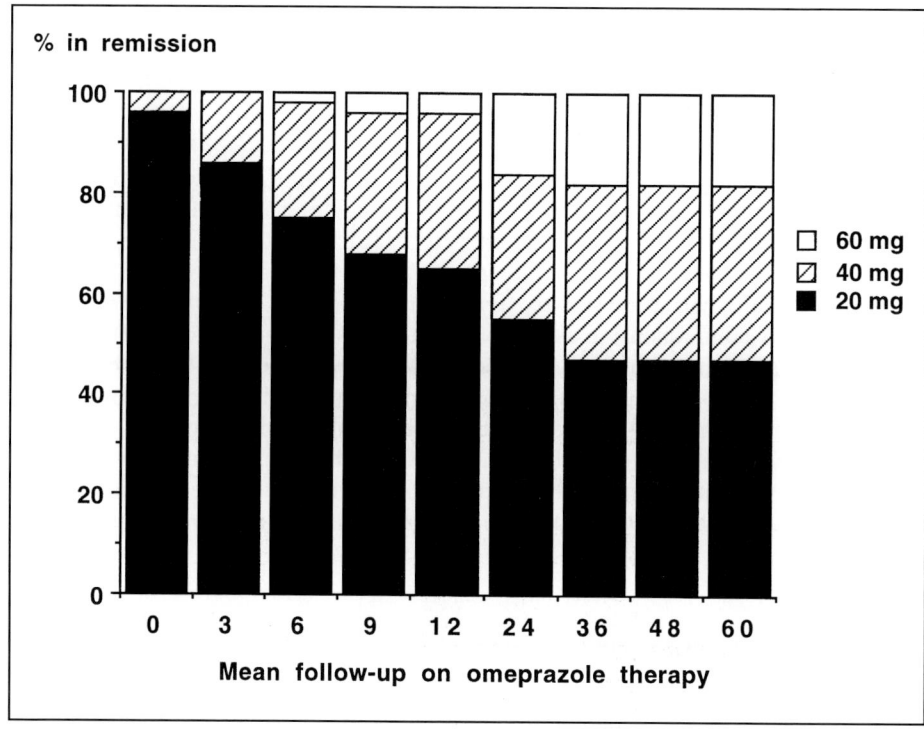

Figure 1. Cumulative remission rates with dose adjustments required to maintain patients with reflux oesophagitis in remission during maintenance treatment with omeprazole. Black bars represent 20 mg daily, hatched bars 40 mg and open bars 60 mg daily.

The natural role of prokinetic agents (the most widely used being cisapride) seems to be in patients with milder forms of the disease, but it should be noted, that a high placebo remission rate has been observed in these trials [19-22]. The initial severity of endoscopic lesions, as well as the type of therapy chosen has a significant impact on the number of patients, who could be kept in remission during maintenance long term therapy [23]. Recent studies have also demonstrated that the presence of Helicobacter pylori infection has a facilitating influence on the efficacy by which proton pump inhibitors can keep these patients in clinical remission [24].

Oesophageal complications of reflux oesophagitis consists primarily of bleeding, ulceration, formation of stricture and the development of columnar lined oesophagus (Barrett's oesophagus). Peptic stricture and Barrett's oesophagus are not only the major, but also the most common serious complications of the disease. The clinical problems related to these manifestations are highly significant and in patients with peptic stricture, the resulting dysphagia can be a major disability that causes nutritional problems. A dilatation of a stricture exposes the patients to a small, but significant risk of oesophageal perforation. Barrett's oesophagus per se really causes morbidity, but carries a significant risk of developing oesophageal adenocarcinoma with its attended morbidity and mortality [25]. The primary, long term aim of medical therapy for patients with peptic stricture and Barrett's oesophagus is the abolition of reflux symptoms and prevention of immediate risk of recurrence or progression of complications. The need for repeated dilatation in patients with peptic stricture is considerably lower in those undergoing fundoplications than in those previously treated conservatively with H_2-receptor antagonits *(figure 2)*. Recent observations with proton pump inhibitors have shown that these drugs have the potential to produce a clinical response very similar to that seen after successful antireflux surgery due to its effects on acid reflux in the oesophagus [26-29].

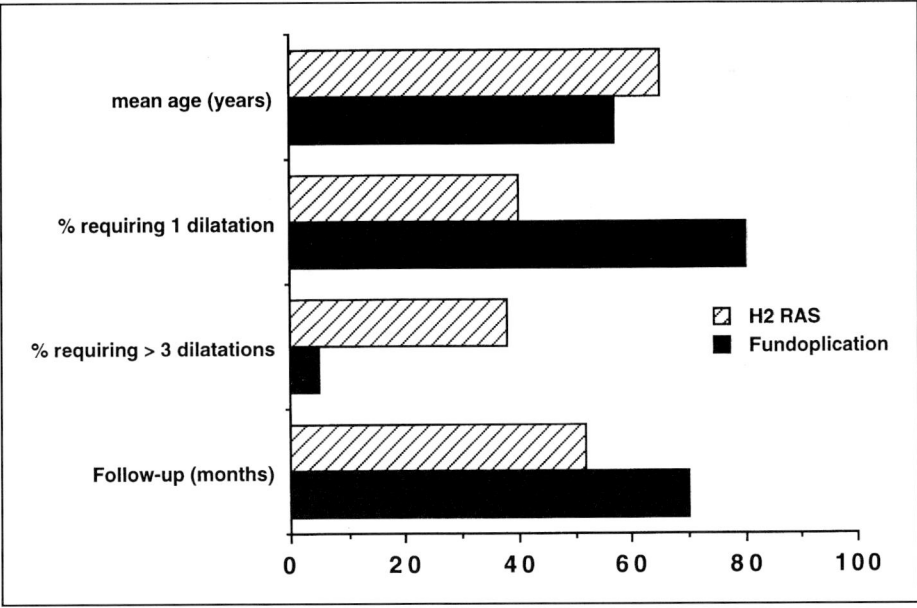

Figure 2. Long term outcome comes of patients with peptic strictures, who were either treated conservatively with antacids or H_2 receptor antagonists (hatched bars) or by antireflux surgery (black bars).

When studying patients with Barrett's oesophagus and the clinical response to different therapeutic interventions, a clear distinction must be made between healing of the oesophagitis and regression of the metaplastic epithelium. A number of reports have been published and demonstrated remarkable symptomatic responses in patients with Barrett's oesophagus when treated with PPIs [30-32]. Similar therapy has not so far been shown to induce any major and significant changes in the length of the columnar lined segment. In addition, it should always be born in mind, that patients with Barrett's oesophagus, in whom reflux is controlled either medically or surgically, must undergo regular surveillance for the development of dysplastic and neoplastic lesions in the metaplastic epithelium [33].

Antireflux surgery

Antireflux surgery is designed to improve the function of the gastro-oesophageal junction and to provide the GORD patients' complete relief of all symptoms and complications of reflux diseases, all of which occur secondary to deficiencies in the reflux preventing barrier located in that area [34, 35]. Ideally, reconstruction of the physiology of the gastro-oesophageal junction should also permit the patients to swallow normally, belch to relieve distension, but hardly to vomit. A major effect of fundoplication operations has been shown to be a substantial reduction in the number of transient lower oesophageal sphincter relaxations [34]. In addition, the proportion of these relaxations accompanied by reflux is decreased, as well as a concomitant increase in the residual pressure at the gastro-oesophageal junction during sphincter relaxation [36, 37]. This is probably another additionally important mechanism to prevent reflux especially in cases with severe complication of the disease. Previous data have repeatedly shown, that fundoplication operations restrain the oesophagal sphincter relaxations to water swallows by what seems to be a purely mechanical effect. The mechanisms by which fundoplications interfere with the triggering of transient sphincter relaxations has, however, yet to be defined. The prevention of reflux during complete lower oesophageal sphincter relaxation, even after fundoplication, suggests that there are other effects of fundoplication on sphincter function separate from that of a simple external cuff. *In vitro* and *in vivo* studies have shown that a sphincter length contributes a sphincter competence and that fundoplication increases the length of the sphincter exposed to intra-abdominal pressure [38, 39]. Undoubtedly, these operations also produce a simple, one-way mechanical flap or flutter valve. Surgical attention has originally focused on the anatomical defects in the hiatus in form of the hernia rather than the problem of physiological defect of incompetence in the reflux preventing mechanisms within the gastro-oesophageal junction. Nissen [40] discovered that the fundic wrap prevented reflux when he studied the patients many years after partial oesophagectomy. Fundoplication has subsequently became the most widely used form of antireflux surgery and the efficacy has been established by clinical and endoscopic follow-up and also by oesophageal 24 hour pH-monitoring, irrespective whether it is performed by an open, conventional technique or by use modern, recently introduced laparoscopic technology [41]. Under the decades, a number of modifications of the original fundoplication operations have evoked, but not every surgeon using the actual technique is as satisfied with the clinical outcome as the originator. On compiling data from controlled, clinical trials it can be concluded that obvious clinical differences in the efficacy between different antireflux procedures seem not to be prevailing, when the outcome is judged with regard to the cumulative GORD relapse rate [42-50]. Excellent control of gastro-oesophageal reflux symptoms can be obtained with the total fundic wrap, a 270° fundoplication, a 180° fundoplication provided that each operation involves the reduction of hiatal hernia coupled with the construction of the valve mechanism to re-establish gastro-oesophageal competence. It must be emphasised that these success rates can and should be achieved with negligable mortality and morbidity. The problem is, however, that published results usually represent the best results in the field of antireflux surgery and the local level of expertise can vary considerably [51, 52]. Accordingly, it is reasonable to propose that antireflux surgery should be performed only in centres, where the expertise has been assembled in the management of gastro-oesophageal reflux disease as well as in the essential diagnostic facilities. Data are accumulating to show that the outcome after laparoscopic fundoplication is as advantageous as that following open surgery [53].

Although antireflux surgery is generally very effective in controlling gastro-oesophageal reflux, some failures are proven unavoidable [54-58]. Persistent postprandial adverse symptoms (in the form of dysphagia, inability to belch and vomit, postprandial fullness, bloating and pain and associally embarrassing rectal flatulence), can mar an otherwise excellent result in a small, but significant group of patients after similar procedures. The frequency by which these postfundoplication symptoms have been reported varies considerably between series, from as low as 0% up to 40%. Dyphagia is frequently reported during the early postoperative period, but vanishes with the passage of time. It should be emphasised that patients very often rate their postprandial symptoms as of doubtful clinical significance and very much less than the preoperative reflux symptoms. Another significant clinical observation is that postfundoplication symptoms, as well as gas-bloat symptoms, improve with the passage of time. Since we lack effective treatment, of established, severe postfundoplication symptoms, prevention is a primary concern. A number of technical considerations have been focused on and alleged to counteract some of these problems, but it must be concluded, based on data from controlled, randomised clinical trials, that as yet no significant differences with regard to postfundoplication symptoms have been firmly established among different antireflux procedures [59]. There is a widespread consensus among experienced surgeons, that if a complete, 360° wrap is done, it has to be both floppy and short, which means that the gastric fundus has to be widely mobilised and that the fundoplication is done only 1 cm long [60, 61]. However, a large randomised clinical trial has reported the semifundoplication according to Toupet to be associated with less troublesome complaints of gas-bloat - rectal flatus [62].

Failure of the fundoplication to control reflux symptoms occurs in 4 to 9% of patients *(figure 3)*. There are reports with a considerably higher failure rate and it is important to emphasise that essentially all failures occur early in the postoperative period, indicating the importance of adhering to techical details.

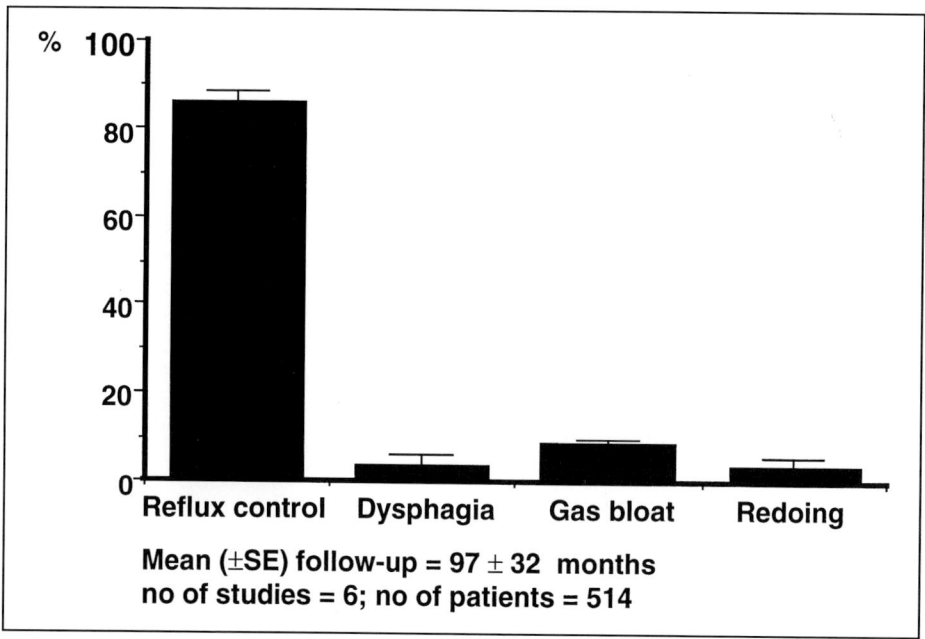

Figure 3. Cumulative remission rates after antireflux surgery when assessed in well controlled clinical trials with long term follow-up.

Comparative trials

The only scientifically effective way of establishing an eventual advantage of one therapeutic principle over another is to carry out comparative, randomised clinical trials. There are a number of obstacles that make the design and logistics of similar trials complicated. Some studies have, however, already been completed, showing an outcome in favour of the surgical alternative [63, 64]. It is interesting to note, that in the Veteran Administration study, the total frequency of complaints was fairly similar in the surgical and medical treatment groups. In the medical arm, the complaints of reflux nature were dominating, whereas in the surgical group post-fundoplication symptoms of varying severity seemed to be most predominating. The problem with this study is the fact that the medical therapy instituted is only historically interesting. In a recently presented, long term follow-up of patients randomised either to omeprazole or antireflux surgery [63], with a minimal follow-up of 3 years, an advantage of antireflux surgery was demonstrated, when 20 mg daily of omeprazole was compared to open antireflux surgery. However, if a dose adjustment was accepted to control symptoms the cumulative relapse rate was identical in the two study arms. Again an advantage was noted in the quality of life assessment in certain dimensions focusing on reflux associated symptoms in the surgical arm, which was compensated for by more indigestion complaints ending up with a fairly similar total score in important quality of life dimensions in the two treatment groups.

It could also be shown that quality of life was normalised already 2 months after initiation of therapy and was thereafter maintained for the years of study.

Although a formal comparison has hitherto not been carried out between modern medical therapy and laparoscopic antireflux surgery, there are no reasons to believe that the outcome of laparoscopic antireflux surgery should be better than that after open procedures [53, 64]. Consequently, the results of the available trials can be extrapolated and have a bearing on the outcome of modern surgical approaches. The great advantage with the surgical procedure is the restoration of the physiology of the gastro-oesophageal junction and the permanent control of all types of reflux with a well documented prospect for the majority of patients to require no further medication. The great disadvantages with the surgical alternative is the safety issue. Although postoperative mortality is exceedingly low, is has to be taken into consideration in patients with a perdefinition, benign disease. The adverse consequences of antireflux surgery are discussed in detail above and also the quality control with to it associated learning curve has to be appreciated. Furthermore, the dependency of the procedures on the skill of the operating surgeon has to be focused on. These pros and cons have to be weighed against pros and cons with medical therapy. The most prominent cons of the latter are; that available effective medical therapy does not affect the deficiencies of the reflux preventing mechanisms, that medical therapy only selectively controls the acid components of the refluxate [65] and that acid inhibition interferes with the gastric milieu, the long term consequences of which have to be determined. In the choice between laparoscopic antireflux surgery and long term proton pump inhibitor therapy these different aspects have to be paid attention to, but of course the preferences of each individual patient has their greatest significance. In young patients with chronic GORD medical therapy is a life long commitment, why the cumulative costs of drugs are essentially out of control compared to the moderate cost associated with laparoscopic antireflux surgery and to it associated rapid recovery [66, 67].

References

1. Olbe L, Lundell L. Medical treatment of reflux esophagitis. *Hepatogastroenterol* 1992; 39: 322-4.
2. Armstrong D, Nicolet M, Monnier T, *et al*. Maintenance therapy: Is there still a place for antireflux surgery? *World J Surg* 1992; 6: 300.
3. Tytgat GNJ, Nio CU, Schotborgh RH. Reflux esophagitis. *Scand J Gastroenterol* 1990; 25 (Suppl. 175): 1.
4. Bell JIV, Hunt RH. Role of gastric acid suppression in the treatment of gastroesophageal reflux disease. *Gut* 1992; 33: 118-24.
5. Bell NJV, Burget D, Howden CW, Wilkinson J, Hunt RH. Appropriate acid suppression for the management of gastroesophageal reflux disease. *Digestion* 1992; 51 (Suppl. 1): 59-67.
6. Van Trappen G, Rutgeer TSL, Schurmans P, Coenegrachts JL. Omeprazole (40 mg) is superior to ranitidine in the short term treatment of ulcerative reflux esophagitis. *Dig Dis Sci* 1988; 33: 523.

7. Sandmark S, Carlsson R, Fausa O, Lundell L. Omeprazole or ranitidine in the treatment of reflux esophagitis. Results of double-blind, randomized, Scandinavian multicenter study. *Scand J Gastroenterol* 1988; 23: 625.
8. Havelund T, Laursen LS, Skoubo-Kristensen E, *et al.* Omeprazole and ranitidine in treatment of reflux esophagitis: double blind comparative trial. *Br Med J* 1988; 296: 89.
9. Klinkenberg-Knol EC, Jansen JBMJ, Festen HPM, Meuwissen SGM, Lamers CBHW. Double blind multicentre comparison of omeprazole and ranitidine in the treatment of reflux esophagitis. *Lancet* 1987; 1: 349.
10. Klinkenberg-Knol EC, Jansen JBMJ, Lamers CBHW, *et al.* Use of omeprazole in the management of reflux esophagitis resistant to H_2-receptor antagonists. *Scand J Gastroenterol* 1989; 24 (Suppl. 166): 88-93.
11. Hetzel DJ, Dent J, Reed WD, *et al.* Healing and relapse of severe peptic esophagitis after treatment with omeprazole. *Gastroenterology* 1988; 95: 903-12.
12. Staerk-Laursen LS, Havelund T, Bondesen S, *et al.* Omeprazole in the long term treatment of gastro-oesophageal reflux disease. A double-blind randomized dose finding study. *Scand J Gastroenterol* 1995; 30: 839-46.
13. Sontag S, Robinson M, Roufail W, *et al.* Daily omeprazole surpasses intermittent dosing in preventing relapse of esophagitis: A US multicenter double-blind study. *Aliment Pharmacol Ther* 1997; 11: 373-80.
14. Hallerbäck B, Unge P, Carling L, *et al.* Omeprazole or ranitidine in long-term treatment of reflux esophagitis. *Gastroenterology* 1994; 107: 1305-11.
15. Dent J, Yeomans ND, Mackinnon M, *et al.* Omeprazole *versus* ranitidine for prevention of relapse in reflux oesophagitis. A controlled double-blind trial of the efficacy and safety. *Gut* 1994; 35: 590-8.
16. Bate CM, Booth SN, Crowe JP, *et al.* Omeprazole 10 mg or 20 mg once daily in the prevention of recurrence of reflux oesophagitis. *Gut* 1995; 36: 492-8.
17. Vigneri S, Termini R, Leandro G, *et al.* A comparison of maintenance therapies for reflux esophagitis. *N Engl J Med* 1995; 333: 1106-10.
18. Lundell L, Backman L, Ekström P, *et al.* Prevention of relapse and reflux esophagitis after endoscopic healing: The efficacy and safety of omeprazole compared with ranitidine. *Scand J Gastroenterol* 1991; 26: 246-56.
19. Koelz HR. Treatment of reflux esophagitis with H_2-blockers, antacids and prokinetic drugs. An analysis of randomised clinical trials. *Scand J Gastroenterol* 1989; 24 (Suppl. 156): 25-36.
20. Tytgat GNJ, Anker-Hansen OJ, Carling L, *et al.* Effect of cisapride on relapse of reflux esophagitis, healed with an antisecretory drug. *Scand J Gastroenterol* 1992; 27: 175-83.
21. Blum AL and the EUROCIS-trialist. Cisapride reduces the relapse rate on reflux esophagitis. World Congress of Gastroenterology, Sydney, Australia 1990.
22. Galmiche JP, Barthelemy P, Hamelin B. Treating the symptoms of gastroesophageal reflux disease. A double-blind comparison of omeprazole and cisapride. *Aliment Pharmacol Ther* 1997; 11: 765-73.
23. Carlsson R, Calmiche JP, Dent J, Lundell L, Frison L. Prognostic factors influencing relapse of oesophagitis during maintenance therapy with antisecretory drugs: A meta-analysis of long term omeprazole trials. *Aliment Pharmacol Ther* 1997; 11: 437-82.
24. Carlsson R. Gastroesophageal reflux disease. A study of pathophysiology clinical diagnosis and management. Gothenburg: University of Gothenburg, 1998, 481 p.
25. Dent J, Bremner CG, Collen MJ, Haggitt RC, Spechler SJ. Working party report to the World Congress of Gastroenterology, Sidney 1990. Barrett's esophagus. *J Gastroenterol Hepatol* 1990; 6: 1-22.
26. Lundell L. Acid suppression in the long-term treatment of peptic stricture and Barrett's esophagus. *Digestion* 1992; 51 (Suppl. 1):49-58.

27. Swarbrick ET, Gough AL, Foster CS, et al. Prevention of recurrence of oesophageal stricture, a comparison of lansoprazole and high-dose ranitidine. *Eur J Gastroenterol Hepatol* 1996; 8: 431-8.
28. Marks RD, Richter JE, Rizzo J, et al. Omeprazole *versus* H_2-receptor antagonists in treating patients with peptic stricture and esophagitis. *Gastroenterology* 1994; 106: 907-15.
29. Smith PM, Kerr GD, Cockel R, et al. A comparison of omeprazole and ranitidine in the prevention of recurrence of benign esophageal stricture. *Gastroenterology* 1994; 107: 1312-8.
30. Deviere J, Buset M, Dumonceau JM, Rickaert F, Cremer M. Regression of Barrett's epithelium with omeprazole. *N Engl J Med* 1989; 320: 1497-8.
31. Gore ES, Healey CJ, Sutton R, Shepherd NA, Wilkinson SP. Regression of columnar lined (Barrett's) esophagus with continuous omeprazole therapy. *Gastroenterology* 1992; 102: A75.
32. Sampliner RE. Antireflux surgery and Barrett's esophagus regression: Wheel or fortune or to tell the truth? *Am J Gastroenterol* 1991; 86: 645-6.
33. Ortiz A, Martinez de Haro LF, Parrilla P, et al. Conservative treatment *versus* antireflux surgery in Barrett's oesophagus: long-term results of a prospective study. *Br J Surg* 1996; 83: 274-8.
34. Ireland AC, Holloway RH, Toouli J, Dent J. Mechanisms underlying the antireflux action of fundoplication. *Gut* 1993; 34: 303.
35. Holloway RH, Dent J. Lower esophageal sphincter dysfunction in gastroesophageal reflux disease. *Gastroenterol Clin N Am* 1990; 19: 517.
36. Bancewicz J, Mughal M, Marples M. The lower esophageal sphincter after floppy Nissen fundoplication. *Br J Surg* 1987; 74: 162.
37. Bjerkeset T, Nordgard K, Schjonsby H. Effect of Nissen fundoplication operation on the competence of the lower esophageal sphincter. *Scand J Gastroenterol* 1980; 15: 213.
38. De Meester TR, Wernly JA, Brian GH, et al. Clinical and *in vitro* analysis of determinants of gastroesophageal competence: A study of the principles of antireflux surgery. *Am J Surg* 1979; 137: 39.
39. Little AG. Mechanism of action of antireflux surgery: theory and facts. *World J Surg* 1992; 16; 320.
40. Nissen R. Eine einfache Operation zur Be-einflussung der Refluxösophagitis. *Schw Med Wochenschr* 1956; 86: 590.
41. Lundell L. The knife or the pill in the long-term treatment of gastroesophageal reflux disease? *Yale J Biol Med* 1994; 67: 233-46.
42. Johansson J, Johnson F, Joelsson BE, Florén CH, Walther B. Outcome from 5 years after 360° fundoplication for gastroesophageal reflux disease. *Br J Surg* 1993; 80: 46.
43. Lundell L, Abrahamsson H, Ruth M, Sandberg N, Olbe L. Lower esophageal sphincter characteristics and esophageal acid exposure following partial or 360° fundoplication: Results of a prospective, randomized, clinical study. *World J Surg* 1991; 15: 115.
44. De Meester TR, Johnson LF, Kent AH. Evaluation of current operations for the prevention of gastroesophageal reflux. *Ann Surg* 1974; 180: 511.
45. Gear MWL, Gillison EW, Dowling BL. Randomised prospective trial of the Angelchik antireflux prosthesis. *Br J Surg* 1984; 71: 681.
46. Kimiot WA, Kirby RM, Akinola D, Temple G. Prospective randomised trial of Nissen fundoplication and Angelchik prosthesis in the surgical treatment of medically refractory gastroesophageal reflux disease. *Br J Surg* 1991; 78: 1181.
47. Stuart RC, Dawson K, Keeling P, Byrne PJ, Hennessy TPJ. A prospective randomized trial of Angelchik prosthesis *versus* Nissen fundoplication. *Br J Surg* 1989; 76: 86.
48. Thor KBA, Silander T. A long-term randomized prospective trial of the Nissen procedure *versus* a modified Toupet technique. *Ann Surg* 1989; 210: 719.

49. Walker SJ, Holt S, Sanderson CJ, Stoddard CJ. Comparison of Nissen total and Lind partial transabdominal fundoplication in the treatment of gastroesophageal reflux. *Br J Surg* 1992; 79: 410.
50. Washer BF, Gear MWL, Dowling BL, *et al.* Randomised prospective trial of Roux-en-Y duodenal diversion *vs* fundoplication for severe reflux esophagitis. *Br J Surg* 1984; 71: 181.
51. Viljakka M, Luostarinen M, Isolauri J. Incidence of antrireflux surgery in Finland 1988-1993. The influence of proton pump inhibitors and laparoscopic technique. *Scand J Gastroenterol* 1997; 32: 415-8.
52. Sanby R, Arvidsson D, Gustavsson S, Hallgren T. Antireflux surgery in Sweden during 1987-1996: A decade of change. *Gastroenterology* 1998; 114: A275.
53. Perdikis G, Hindler RA, Lund RJ, Raiser F, Katada N. Laparoscopic Nissen fundoplication: Where do we stand? *Surg Laparosc Endosc* 1997; 7: 17-21.
54. Garstin WI, Hohnston GW, Kennedy TL, Spencer ES. Nissen fundoplication: the unhappy 15%. *J R Coll Surg*, Edinburgh, 1986; 31: 207.
55. Negre JB. Post-fundoplication symptoms. Do they restrict the success of Nissen fundoplication? *Ann Surg* 1983; 198: 698.
56. De Meester TR, Stein HJ. Minimizing the side effects of antireflux surgery. *World J Surg* 1992; 16: 335.
57. Mughal MM, Bancewicz J, Marpels M. Oesophageal manometry and pH recording does not predict the bad results of Nissen fundoplication. *Br J Surg* 1990; 77: 43.
58. Siewert RJ, Isolauri J, Feussner H. Reoperation following failed fundoplication. *World J Surg* 1989; 13: 791.
59. Watson A. Update: Total *versus* partial laparoscopic fundoplication. *Dig Surg* 1998; 15: 172-80.
60. Donahue PE, Samuelson S, Nyhus LM, Bombeck CT. The floppy Nissen fundoplication. *Arch Surg* 1985; 120: 663.
61. Dalenbäck J, Lönroth H, Blomqvist A, Lundell L. Improved functional outcome after laparoscopic fundoplication by complete gastric fundus mobilization. *Gastroenterology* 1998; 114: A1384 SSAT Abstracts.
62. Lundell L, Abrahamsson H, Ruth M, Rydberg L, Lönroth H, Olbe L. Long-term results of a prospective randomized comparison of total fundic wrap (Nissen-Rossetti) or semifundoplication (Toupet) for gastro-oesophageal reflux. *Br J Surg* 1996; 83: 830-5.
63. Lundell L, Dalenbäck J, Hattlebakk J, *et al.* Omeprazole (OME) or antireflux surgery (ARS) in the long term management of gastroesophageal reflux disease (GERD): Results of a multicentre, randomised clinical trial. *Gastroenterology* 1998; 114: A207.
64. Behar J, Sheahan DG, Biancani P, Spiro HM, Storer EH. Medical and surgical management of reflux esophagitis. A 38-month report on a prospective clinical trial. *N Engl J Med* 1975; 293: 263-8.
65. Spechler SJ. Comparison of medical and surgical therapy for complicated gastroesophageal reflux disease in veterans. The Department of Veterans Affairs Gastroesophageal Reflux Disease Study Group. *N Engl J Med* 326: 786-92.
66. Peracchia A, Bancewicz J, Bonavina L, *et al.* Fundoplication is an effective treatment for gastro-oesophageal reflux disease. *Gastroenterol Int* 1995; 8: 1-7.
67. Blomqvist AMK, Lönroth H, Dalenbäck J, Lundell L. Laparoscopic or open fundoplication? A complete cost analysis. *Surg Endosc* 1998, in press.
68. Myrvold HE, Lundell L, Liedman B, *et al.* The cost of omeprazole *versus* open anti-reflux surgery in the long-term management of reflux esophagitis. *Gastroenterology* 1998; 114: A238.

Progress in functional disorders

Functional disorders of the upper gastrointestinal tract.
New concepts

R.H. Hunt, E.L. Fallen, M.V. Kamath, A.R.M. Upton, G. Tougas

Divisions of Gastroenterology and Cardiology, Department of Medicine, McMaster University Medical Centre, Hamilton, Ontario L8N 3Z5, Canada

Functional gastrointestinal disorders are common and may be generalized or localized either to the upper or lower GI tract. In the upper GI tract, symptoms including those of dyspepsia (non-ulcer dyspepsia (NUD) and non-cardiac chest pain (NCCP) has been more extensively studied.

Historically, these conditions have been thought to originate from some disorder of gut motility, and indeed, many patients are found to have some degree of altered motility, when assessed using manometry, radiology or scintigraphy. Investigators have also used newer techniques such as ultrasound, electrogastrography, magnetic resonance imaging (MRI), barostat, etc. to measure gastric emptying, luminal transit, myoelectrical disturbances, or visceral tone and perception. More recently, we, and others, have developed new approaches to assessing both afferent and efferent aspects of the gut brain axis and established the gut brain cardiac responses as a parameter of visceral response to gut stimulation. This provides the opportunity to speculate on novel aspects of visceral perception in functional disorders of the upper GI tract.

Dyspepsia and non-cardiac chest pain

While recognizing dyspepsia as a multi-component, multi-faceted disorder which may incorporate reflux like, ulcer like, and dysmotility like symptoms, no obvious cause(s) have been identified. Moreover, many patients do not show any evidence of abnormality even when investigated by an extensive battery of tests such as those listed above. Indeed, even when abnormalities are demonstrated, treatment of motor abnormalities may not result in any improvement in symptoms. Furthermore, there is no clear association between the presence of structural abnormalities, such as gastritis and symptoms, and the eradication of *H. pylori* infection with gastritis resolution of has produced, at best, variable results in clinical trials.

The concept of visceral hypersensitivity has been proposed as one way of explaining such confusing findings. Most patients with functional upper GI disorders, such as NUD or NCCP, report pain from mechanical (balloon distention) or chemical stimulation (HCl perfusion) of the esophagus or stomach at significantly lower levels than healthy subjects, suggesting that allodynia and/or hyperalgesia may be present.

In non-cardiac chest pain, gastroenterologists have increasingly been attracted to the idea of esophageal causes as the source for the symptoms. Patients often report atypical features of pain, which may include severe intensity, prolonged duration and a variable response to anti-anginal therapy. In most patients with NCCP, cardiac studies are negative in the majority of patients, together with normal coronary artery angiograms, including those who may present with some mild features of ischemia on ECG, suggesting that they have exaggerated or abnormal cardiac pain perception. This condition has been designated as Syndrome X and is associated with abnormal endothelial function, and excessive sympathetic drive or responsiveness.

Gut-brain-gut communications

Studies of the gut-brain-gut communications and connections are in their infancy but sophisticated methods are becoming increasingly available. Recent work from our group has shown that balloon inflation or electrical stimulation in the esophagus is associated with predictable and reproducible cerebral evoked responses, a finding subsequently confirmed also by others. The velocity of the afferent impulse differs according to transmission either *via* slow C fibers with balloon distention, or faster, myelinated A delta fibers in response to electrical stimulation. It is now possible to determine the effect of visceral afferent sensory stimuli originating from the gastrointestinal tract on the autonomic efferent output elicited by the brain in response to the sensory stimulus. In our laboratory, we use power spectral analysis of the beat to beat heart rate variability to determine the impact of visceral sensory stimuli on efferent autonomic outflow to the heart. Balloon or electrical stimulation from the esophagus produces marked and opposing alterations in the respective magnitude of the low and high frequency peaks present in the power spectral distribution of heart rate variability, reflecting a simultaneous decrease in sympathetic cardiac outflow and increase in the parasympathetic (vagal) cardiac tone.

In NCCP patients, we have shown that non-cardiac chest pain patients who have a high resting sympathetic tone are much more likely (probability > 95%) to develop symptoms of chest pain in response to esophageal acid perfusion, than in those in whom the resting vagal peak is dominant.

These techniques and other similar approaches now offer the opportunity to study functional disorders of the gastrointestinal tract in a more objective manner than has previously been possible. Indeed, our findings indicate that a spectrum of afferent stimuli arising from the gut or other sensory apparatus may alter efferent autonomic function and modify the relative influence of the sympathetic and parasympathetic nervous systems on visceral organs.

Conceptually, this offers an intriguing opportunity to hypothesize on the origins for a variety of functional gastrointestinal disorders as well as other conditions such as labile hypertension, non-allergic bronchospasm, fibromyalgia, fibromyosytis, etc.

Visceral sensations are transmitted either *via* afferent nervous fibers in the vagus or through spinal afferent pathways with cell bodies in the dorsal root ganglia, which project to the dorsal horn of the spinal cord. From the dorsal horn, higher order neurons transmit to the brainstem and thalamus, with subsequent impulses eventually reaching the cerebral cortex where conscious perception occurs.

So how might alterations in afferent neural signaling arise in patients with functional upper GI tract disorders?

Inflammation in the GI tract

A number of possible mechanisms involving the enteric nervous system and the central nervous system may be disordered in dyspeptic patients or NCCP patients. Recent concepts concerning the role of inflammation leading to dysfunction in the intestine may also be relevant to the role of *H. pylori* in patients with dyspepsia. Modification of afferent signaling might occur as a result of inflammation resulting from *H. pylori* infection. A model for this comes from the evidence that the stimulus - response curve to distention of the bladder is shifted in the presence of bladder inflammation and this is associated with the recruitment of new afferent fibers. The release of cytokines in response to mucosal inflammation also can lead to the release of IL-1β, which has been shown to excite neurons and increase pain perception, by the release of mucosal prostanoids. The alteration of nor-adrenaline release in models of intestinal inflammation also may result from the release of cytokines in the mucosa. The release of neuropeptides such as somatostatin and substance P may also lead to changes in myenteric nerve function. In addition, there is evidence that *H. pylori* infection is associated with remodeling of mucosal nerves as a result of the inflammatory process. More recent work from our group has reported changes in immunoreactive staining of substance P and CRGP containing nerves in the dorsal horn of the spinal cord in experimental *Helicobacter* infection in rodents.

Basal sympathetic and parasympathetic activity

As a consequence of changes in afferent stimulation or perception, central perception may be altered and lead to altered efferent output resulting in abnormal stimulation or function of the gastrointestinal tract. An excellent model to study such events in animals is the Flinders strain of rats, which includes the Flinders Sensitive Line (FSL) and the Flinders Resistant Line (FSR). The FSL is a strain of rat, which is known to exhibit low basal vagal activity and marked cholinergic hyper-sensitivity. This is associated with an excessive vagal responsiveness to external and internal stimuli. Its normal counterpart is the FRL line rat. Like it has previously been shown in normal Sprague Dawley rats, both strains respond to gastric distention with a volume dependent decrease in heart rate, which is a physiological response that mirrors the intensity of the perceived visceral sensory stimulus (pseudo-affective response). This response is vagally mediated and abolished by prior atropine or subdiaphragmatic vagotomy. In the presence of intestinal inflammation induced by *T. spiralis* infection the response is markedly altered, with an increased response in the cholinergic sensitive animal (the FSL) and a decreased response in the control counterpart. This decreased response is identical to the previously described response in Sprague Dawley rats with *T. spiralis* infection. The increased responsiveness seen in the cholinergic sensitive line is the same as occurs in patients with esophageal acid sensitivity, as described above. This observation reinforces the concept that the underlying autonomic function is an important modulator of visceral sensitivity, with a low resting vagal tone and high resting sympathetic tone, as seen in the FSL animals, and in NCCP patients. Both in NCCP patients and in Flinders rats, it is only if the resting vagal tone is low that there will be an excessive vagal response to a visceral stimulus, which in humans is associated with increased pain in response to a visceral stimulus. In the same Flinders Strain model the effect of stress can be studied. Stress is produced by mild restraint for 2 hours prior to the animals being studied in the same manner as above, with the cardiac response to gastric distention producing volume dependent vagally mediated decreases in heart rate. In the unstressed situation, the FSL and FRL rats both show a normal response (as do normal, unstressed Sprague Dawley rats). However, following the restraint stress, the cardiac response to gastric distention is markedly enhanced in the FSL rats, but not in FRL or Sprague Dawley rats. This implies that stress, like inflammation in the *T. spiralis* model, induces an acute hyperalgesia in the FSL animal, similar to what is often seen in humans.

Stress has long been thought to be important in functional disorders of the gut and modifies the immune response both concurrently and at a point distant in time. More recently, mental activity has been shown to modulate gut perception, with significantly increased perception observed during attention when compared to distraction.

Conclusion

Thus, new techniques for investigating the afferent nervous system and an increasing understanding of the role of increased visceral hypersensitivity is leading to broader concepts of the origins and mechanisms involved in functional disease of the upper GI tract.

Bibliography

1. Accarino AM, Azpiroz F, Malagelada JR. Attention and distraction: effects on gut perception. *Gastroenterology* 1997; 113: 415-22.
2. Armstrong D, Spaziani RM, Fallen EL, Kamath MV, Collins SM, Tougas G. Barostat controlled esophageal balloon distension produces a pressure-dependent heart rate decrease in healthy subjects. *Gastroenterology* 1996; 110: A624.
3. Bennett EJ, Piesse C, Palmer K, Badcock CA, Tennant CC, Kellow JE. Functional gastrointestinal disorders: psychological, social, and somatic features. *Gut* 1998; 42 (3): 414-20.
4. Cannon RO. Chest pain and the sensitive heart. *Eur J Gastroenterol Hepatol* 1995; 7: 1166-71.
5. Cannon RO, Benjamin SB. Chest pain as a consequence of abnormal visceral nociception. *Dig Dis Sci* 1993; 38: 193-6.
6. Collins SM, Hurst SM, Main C, et al. Effect of inflammation of enteric nerves. Cytokine induced changes in neurotransmitter content and release. *Ann NY Acad Sci* 1992; 664: 415-24.
7. Collins SM, Blennerhassett P, Degiorgio R, Barbara G, Tougas G, Li H, Larsson H. The impact of *Helicobacter pylori* infection on gastric neuromuscular function in the rat; basic observations and clinical implications for our understanding of functional dyspepsia. In: Hunt RH, Tytgat GNJ, eds. Helicobacter pylori: *basic mechanisms to clinical cure*. Dordrecht: Kluwer, 1998: 195-205.
8. Holtmann G, Goebell H, Jockenhoevel F, Talley NJ. Altered vagal and intestinal mechanosensory function in chronic unexplained dyspepsia. *Gut* 1998; 42 (4): 501-6.
9. Hollerbach S, Kamath MV, Chen Y, Fitzpatrick D, Upton AR, Tougas G. The magnitude of the central response to esophageal electrical stimulation is intensity dependent. A dose-response study. *Gastroenterology* 1997; 112 (4): 1137-46.
10. Jacobson K, McHugh K, Collins SM. Experimental colitis alters myenteric nerve function at inflamed and non-inflamed sites in the rat. *Gastroenterology* 1995; 109: 718-22.
11. Mayer EA, Raybould H, Koelbel C. Neuropeptides, inflammation, and motility. *Dig Dis Sci* 1988; 33: 71S-7S.
12. Mayer EA, Raybould H. Role of visceral afferent mechanisms in functional bowel disorders. *Gastroenterology* 1990; 99: 1688-704.
13. McMahon SB, Koltzenburg M. Changes in the afferent innervation of the inflamed urinary bladder. In: Meyer EA, Raybould HE, eds. *Basic and clinical aspects of chronic abdominal pain*. Amsterdam: Elsevier, 1993: 155-72.
14. Sridhar S, Djuric V, Spaziani R, Kamath M, Armstrong D, Fallen E, Upton A, Tougas G. Esophageal sensitivity and autonomic response to acid perfusion in patients with non-cardiac chest pain. *Can J Gastroenterol* 1996; 10 (Suppl. A): 11A(F69).
15. Spaziani RM, Djuric V, Kamath MV, et al. A low resting vagal tone predicts response to acid perfusion in patients with esophageal symptoms. *Gastroenterology* 1996; 110: A762.
16. Stead RH, Hewlett BR, Lhotak S, Colley ECC, Frendo M, Dixon MF. Do gastric mucosal nerves re-model in *H. pylori* gastritis? In: Hunt RH, Tytgat GNJ, eds. Helicobacter pylori: *basic mechanisms to clinical cure*. Dordrecht: Kluwer, 1994: 281-91.
17. Talley NJ, Hunt RH. What role does *Helicobacter pylori* play in dyspepsia and non-ulcer dyspepsia? Arguments for and against *H. pylori* being associated with dyspeptic symptoms. *Gastroenterology* 1997; 113 (6 Suppl.): S67-77.
18. Tougas G, Hudoba P, Fitzpatrick D, Hunt RH, Upton AR. Cerebral-evoked potential responses following direct vagal and esophageal electrical stimulation in humans. *Am J Physiol* 1993; 264: G486-91.
19. Tougas G, Kamath M, Watteel G, Fitzpatrick D, Fallen EL, Hunt RH, Upton AR. Modulation of neurocardiac function by oesophageal stimulation in humans. *Clin Sci* 1997; 92: 167-74.

20. Vermillion DL, Ernst PB, Scicchitano R, Collins SM. Antigen-induced contraction of jejunal smooth muscle in the sensitized rat. *Am J Physiol* 1988; 255: G701-8.
21. Wang L, Chen Y, Djuric V, Steiner M, Overstreet DH, Tougas G. Acute stress increases the vagal response to gastric distention (GD) in a rat model of cholinergic hypersensitivity. *Gastroenterology* 1998; 114 (4): G3517.
22. Wang L, Djuric V, Blennerhassett PA, Steiner M, Overstreet DH, Collins SM, Tougas G. Increased worm expulsion and vagal response to gastric distention (GD) following *T. Spiralis* infection in a rat model of cholinergic hyper-responsiveness. *Gastroenterology* 1998; 114 (4): G3519.

Progress in functional disorders: functional lower intestinal disease

E.A. Mayer

UCLA School of Medicine, Los Angeles, CA 90024, USA

Evolving disease model – alterations in brain-gut interactions

In contrast to the reductionistic disease models of the past, which have included psychiatric, inflammatory and motility versions, IBS and related functional disorders are now being viewed as clinical manifestations of alterations in the bidirectional communication between the digestive, the immune and the nervous systems. These alterations manifest as aberrant gastrointestinal motor responses to stress and food intake [1], as enhanced perceptual responses to visceral stimuli, as prolonged mucosal abnormalities following gastroenteric infections, and in a subset of patients as affective symptoms.

A number abnormal motor patterns have been reported by different investigators in patients with IBS. These patterns are non-specific, also occur in healthy subjects and rarely correlate with symptoms suggesting that these reported motility alterations are a secondary phenomena rather than a primary etiologic factor in IBS. Several studies have shown hypermotility of the rectosigmoid colon in response to eating or laboratory stressors which may explain why many patients with IBS experience typical IBS symptoms after meals or develop exacerbation of symptoms during stressful life events.

The lack of correlation between symptoms and abnormal intestinal motility has resulted in a refocusing of research efforts into identifying alterations in the perception of visceral events as a cause of the most typical IBS symptoms, such as abdominal pain and bloating-type symptoms. In contrast to other physiologic mechanisms proposed to explain symptom generation in IBS patients, alterations in the processing of viscero-sensory information has been the most reproducible marker of this disorder to date. Several studies have reported that IBS patients report discomfort and pain at lower distention intensities when balloons are inflated throughout the gastrointestinal tract. These findings do not appear to be secondary to alterations in intestinal tone or compliance, nor do they correlate with measures of psychoneuroticism. IBS patients do appear to be more vigilant towards potentially aversive visceral sensations [2], show alterations in viscerosomatic referral [3] and demonstrate a unique hyperalgesic response to repetitive distension of the sigmoid colon [4]. Consistent with the reported alterations in the perception of visceral afferent information, specific alterations in regional brain activation have recently been reported in IBS patients [5].

Multicomponent disease model for FDD

While neither the reported alterations in GI motility or visceral sensation by themselves explain the full clinical presentation of IBS, a multicomponent model of IBS, similar to other chronic illnesses, involving physiologic, affective, cognitive, and behavioral factors, can be formulated. The importance of each factor in the generation of IBS symptoms may vary between person to person.

- **Behavioral factors** such as stressful life events are reported by up to 60% of IBS patients to be associated with the first onset of symptoms or with its symptom exacerbation [6].

- **Cognitive factors** such as inappropriate coping styles, illness behavior and inappropriate concepts about disease, nutrition and medications are common in IBS patients. These factors in turn determine the response to and coping with stressors, either related to symptoms or to stressful life events. Cognitive factors have a prominent influence on healthcare utilization and clinical outcomes.

- **Affective factors**, such as anxiety and depression, are present in a large percentage of IBS patients seeking healthcare, primarily in the form of anxiety, panic disorder and depression.

- **Physiologic factors** implicated in the generation of IBS symptoms include hypersensitivity of the GI tract to normal events, autonomic dysfunction including altered intestinal motility response to stress, anger, and food intake, changes in fluid and electrolyte processing by the bowel, altered responses of the hypothalamic-pituitary-adrenal (HPA) axis and alterations in sleep [7].

Etiologic model for FDD

Current evidence is consistent with an etiologic model for FDD which assumes a predisposition of the nervous system in addition to specific environmental trigger factors. The predisposition may occur in form of genetic factors or in form of early life events, including perinatal events. The trigger factors may occur in form of psychosocial stressors or in form of physical stressors (gastroenteric infection, inflammation, tissue irritation).

Genetic factors

Recent data suggest that genetic predisposition may contribute to the development of IBS in some patients. Symptoms consistent with IBS are more common in first degree relatives but not spouses of subjects with IBS. Additionally, in a study of twin pairs in Australia, a proportion of the incidence of IBS in both twins was felt to be due to genetic rather than environmental factors. Further studies are needed to differentiate the effect of parent behavior and family environment from that of genetic factors.

Perinatal events

Perinatal events may play a role in altering the nervous system in a way that makes the individual more sensitive to internal events and more prone to central dysregulation of intestinal motor and secretory function. The nervous system is more vulnerable during pre- and early postnatal period to perturbations, and changes occurring during this period may have long-lasting effects due to neuroplastic changes in the CNS. Such perinatal events may occur in form of tissue irritation from gastroesophageal reflux disease, intestinal inflammation due to food intolerances and allergies, or they may occur in form of neuroendocrine changes related to stress. Such neuroendocrine correlates of stress may be transmitted from the mother *via* increased cortisol and catecholamine levels in the breast milk, or they may be generated by the newborn itself. Recent animal experimental data has demonstrated profound, longlasting changes in the nervous system in the form of hyperresponsiveness, irritability and predisposition to affective disorders in response to such perinatal stressors.

Chronic psychosocial stressors

Stressful life events are often reported by patients to precede the onset or exacerbation of IBS symptoms. A questionnaire study of 135 patients with IBS and 654 controls, 73% of the IBS and 54% of the control group reported that stress altered their stool pattern, while 84% of the IBS and 68% of the control group reported that stress led to abdominal pain. Stress also correlates with the frequency of bowel symptoms, the number of disability days, and the number of physician visits.

Acute, life threatening stressors (PTSD)

A history of severe emotional trauma such as physical and sexual abuse, especially when incurred during childhood, is associated with an increased risk to develop IBS. In one study at the University of North Carolina, 53% of women with IBS gave a history of abuse in comparison to 37% of women with structural GI diagnoses. However, more recent studies indicate that only acute stressful events associated with a direct threat to an individual's life are associated with a higher incidence of FDD.

Physical stressors

IBS symptoms occur in approximately one-third of patients symptoms following acute GI infections often persisting for years following complete resolution of the infection. On the other hand, only a small percentage of all IBS patients will present such a history. A prospective study found that psychometric scores for anxiety, depression, somatization, and neurotic traits were higher in those individuals who developed prolonged IBS symptoms following their acute gastroenteritis than those patients who later returned to normal bowel function. This suggests that only in predisposed individuals enteric infections and presumably other causes of mucosal irritation can precipitate on-going IBS symptoms which may persist long after the infection (or inflammation) has resolved. The fact that affective disorders appear to be part of this predisposition, is consistent with a role of CNS alterations in the etiology of IBS. Recent evidence suggests that alterations in the neuroendocrine response to stress (both physical and psychosocial stressors) may be one of the underlying mechanism resulting in prolonged proinflammatory mucosal changes in IBS.

Correlation of FDD with psychiatric disorders

Co-morbid psychiatric diagnoses (the most common being depression and generalized anxiety disorder) are present in up 42-61% of patients with IBS referred to a tertiary referral center. The life time prevalence of these disorders in an IBS population reaches 90%. While some studies show that IBS "non-patients", have psychologically characteristics similar to the general population, a recent population-based survey within the US concluded that the prevalence of certain psychiatric diagnoses, such as panic disorder or anxiety are equally common in patients with IBS symptoms, regardless if they have consulted a physician for their symptoms or not (B. Lydiard, personal communication, Sept. 1997). It remains to be determined if this high degree of co-morbidity is a consequence of having a chronic disease which severely impacts quality of life, if it is a random co-occurrence of common disorders, or if the CNS alterations underlying affective disorders and changes in visceral sensory and autonomic regulation affect similar neurophysiological mechanisms. In addition to the high prevalence of affective disorders, many patients with IBS have ineffective coping skills for managing their symptoms and for life stresses in general.

Therapeutic approaches

A number of pharmacological, psychological and alternative therapies are currently being used to treat patients with IBS, however, their efficacy has not been proven. An extensive review of randomized, double-blind, placebo-controlled drug trials performed between 1966 and 1988 by Klein [8] found that none of the studies provided sound statistical evidence to suggest that any of the medications were significantly beneficial in the treating the symptoms of IBS. Most studies were flawed because of short treatment periods (1/2 were less than 4 weeks), poor operational definition of IBS, cross-over design, and a short or no follow-up period [8]. Likewise, a critical review of psychotherapies for IBS by Talley found no one form of therapy to be definitely better than placebo, and most of the studies to be flawed [9]. Despite the lack of reliable controlled outcome data, there is a general consensus that both pharmacological and behavioral approaches can improve specific disease components such as altered bowel habits, abdominal pain and discomfort and affective disease components.

Evolving therapies

In lack of a definitive etiology or pathophysiology, it is difficult to evaluate current and evolving therapies. For example, even though a compound has been developed or is being marketed as an antispasmodic, aimed at a peripheral target to decrease the contractility of smooth muscle, it may exert its therapeutic effect *via* supraspinal muscarinic or antimuscarinic effects on central autonomic control or pain perception. The same argument holds true for compounds aimed at different serotonin receptors, opioid receptors or tricyclic antidepressants. Despite these considerations, it is possible to discuss evolving therapies and those which are in development under two main categories : those aimed at decreasing the transmission of viscerosensory information from the periphery to the brain (assuming a "hypersensitive gut"), and those aimed at decreasing the amplification of viscerosensory information by the brain (assuming a "hypersensitive brain").

Conclusion

Considerable progress has been made within the last 5 years in the conceptualization of pathophysiology and etiology of various functional gastrointestinal disorders, including IBS. While little scientific evidence supports the usefulness of the most commonly prescribed medications for IBS and other functional GI disorders, evolving drug development will allow us to confirm or eliminate scientific hypothesis (hypersensitive gut *vs* hypersensitive brain) and will hopefully provide effective therapies before the end of the century.

References

1. Quigley EMM. Intestinal manometry – technical advances, clinical limitations. *Dig Dis Sci* 1992; 37: 10-3.
2. Naliboff BD, Munakata J, Fullerton S, Gracely RH, Kodner A, Harraf F, Mayer EA. Evidence for two distinct perceptual alterations in irritable bowel syndrome. *Gut* 1997; 41: 505-12.
3. Mertz H, Naliboff B, Munakata J, Niazi N, Mayer E. Altered rectal perception is a biological marker of patients with the irritable bowel syndrome. *Gastroenterology* 1995; 109: 40-52.
4. Munakata J, Naliboff B, Harraf F, Kodner A, Lembo T, Chang L, Silverman DH, Mayer EA. Repetitive sigmoid stimulation induces rectal hyperalgesia in patients with irritable syndrome. *Gastroenterology* 1997; 112 (1): 55-63.
5. Silverman DH, Munakata JA, Ennes H, Mandelkern MA, Hoh CK, Mayer EA. Regional cerebral activity in normal and pathological perception of visceral pain. *Gastroenterology* 1997; 112 (1): 64-72.
6. Whitehead WE, Bosmajian L, Zonderman AB, Costa Jr PT, Schuster MM. Symptoms of psychological distress associated with irritable bowel syndrome. *Gastroenterology* 1988; 95: 709-14.
7. Mayer EA, Gebhart GF. Basic and clinical aspects of visceral hyperalgesia. *Gastroenterology* 1994; 107: 271-93.
8. Klein KB. Controlled treatment trials in the irritable bowel syndrome: a critique. *Gastroenterology* 1988; 95: 232-41.
9. Talley NJ, Owen BK, Boyce P, Paterson K. Psychological treatments for irritable syndrome: a critique of controlled treatment trials. *Am J Gastroenterol* 1996; 91 (2): 277-83.

Achevé d'imprimer par Corlet, Imprimeur, S.A.
14110 Condé-sur-Noireau (France)
N° d'Imprimeur : 32882 - Dépôt légal : août 1998

Imprimé en U.E.